Forever Strong

Forever Strong

A New, Science-Based Strategy for Aging Well

DR. GABRIELLE LYON

ATRIA BOOKS

NEW YORK   LONDON   TORONTO   SYDNEY   NEW DELHI

ATRIA
BOOKS

An Imprint of Simon & Schuster, Inc.
1230 Avenue of the Americas
New York, NY 10020

First Atria Books hardcover edition October 2023

ATRIA BOOKS and colophon are trademarks of Simon & Schuster, Inc.

For information about special discounts for bulk purchases, please contact Simon & Schuster Special Sales at 1-866-506-1949 or business@simonandschuster.com.

The Simon & Schuster Speakers Bureau can bring authors to your live event. For more information or to book an event, contact the Simon & Schuster Speakers Bureau at 1-866-248-3049 or visit our website at www.simonspeakers.com.

Interior design by Timothy Shaner, NightandDayDesign.biz

Manufactured in the United States of America

3 5 7 9 10 8 6 4

Library of Congress Cataloging-in-Publication Data
Names: Lyon, Gabrielle (Osteopath), author.
Title: Forever strong : a new, science-based strategy for aging well / by Gabrielle Lyon.
Description: First Atria Books hardcover edition. | New York : Atria Books, 2023. | Includes bibliographical references.
Identifiers: LCCN 2023016858 (print) | LCCN 2023016859 (ebook) | ISBN 9781668007877 (hardcover) | ISBN 9781668007884 (trade paperback) | ISBN 9781668044445 (trade paperback) | ISBN 9781668007891 (ebook)
Subjects: LCSH: Longevity—Nutritional aspects. | Aging—Prevention. | Muscle strength—Health spects.
Classification: LCC RA776.75 .L96 2023 (print) | LCC RA776.75 (ebook) | DDC 612.6/8--dc23/eng/20230623
LC record available at https://lccn.loc.gov/2023016858
LC ebook record available at https://lccn.loc.gov/2023016859

ISBN 978-1-6680-0787-7
ISBN 978+1-6680-0789-1 (ebook)

Dedicated to my best friend and mentor
of a lifetime, Dr. Donald Layman

CONTENTS

Forever
Strong

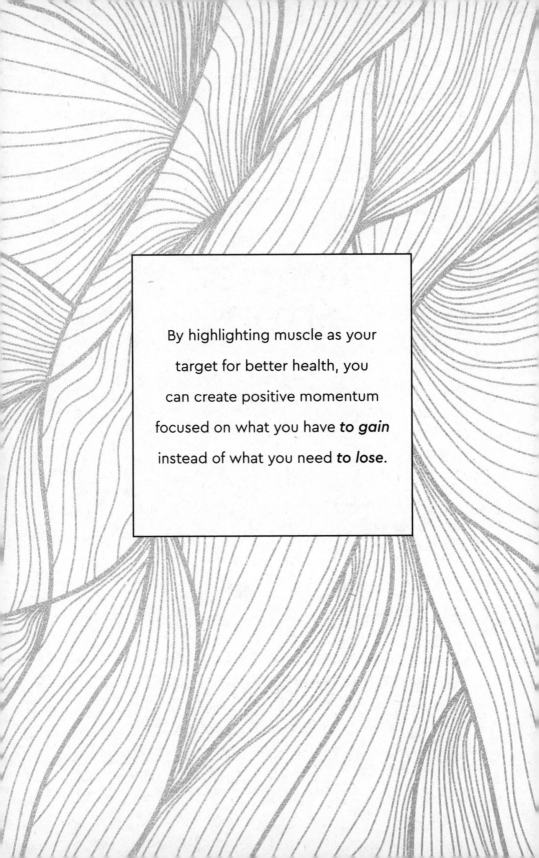

By highlighting muscle as your target for better health, you can create positive momentum focused on what you have *to gain* instead of what you need *to lose*.

Introduction

W hat you are about to read has the power to transform your life. My goal with this book—and with all my work in Muscle-Centric Medicine®—is to overthrow conventional wisdom on the foundation of good health. I want to help you get to the root of where your body's strength lies so you can take swift and effective steps to feel stronger, look better, and add years to your life.

You've already heard that you need to eat right, exercise, and lower your stress level to live longer, right? So why does it feel so difficult to make even the most basic commitments to a healthy life? I believe good health starts with the most important muscle of all: your mind. After I completed med school, I spent two years in psychiatry to study what makes people the best versions of themselves. The thinking patterns and brain pathology I studied have since become invaluable to my work helping patients get well and reach their full potential. And yet, after my transition to family medicine, patients came to me in the prime of their lives already showing signs of type 2 diabetes, cardiovascular disease, and obesity. Still, there seemed to be no room to talk about prevention besides generic recommendations—with limited impact. The chance to provide nutritional counseling as part of my residency, which focused on obesity and weight management, granted me another window into the painful consequences of damaging lifestyle patterns. So many patients felt trapped on a hamster wheel of frustration. I felt just as frustrated by the limits of mainstream medicine.

After my residency, I attended Washington University for a combined research and medical fellowship in geriatrics and nutritional sciences. I engaged with next-level nutrition research in the lab of Dr. Sam Klein, who is known for studying the clinical and metabolic aspects of obesity and type 2 diabetes. For two years, I ran an obesity clinic, sitting week after week with the struggling participants. I witnessed the pain of people trying, unsuccessfully, to lose weight, and it kept haunting me: Why, with all our scientific insights, are we still chasing obesity?

The question felt especially urgent when I attended to my clinical responsibilities as a geriatric fellow providing advanced aging care. Daily, I witnessed the devastation wrought by dementia on patients and their families. The ramifications of that focus for the aging population pained me, but working with these two patient populations helped me connect the dots. This combination of duties revealed to me the before-and-after consequences of nutrition and exercise choices made by individuals who'd been left floundering by flawed recommendations. I also had an even bigger revelation when I discovered that the one thing that both these groups had in common wasn't a "weight problem" but a muscle problem.

One study I worked on examined the connections between body weight and brain function and found a correlation between a wider waistline and lower brain volume. The working premise was that obesity causes insulin resistance in the brain—a sort of "type 3 diabetes" of cerebral matter—that could lead to dementia. Our research showed that people with obesity often had impaired overall cognitive responses, such as impulse control, task switching, and other mental challenges.[1] I became very invested in the study's participants, especially Betsy, a mother of three in her early fifties, who had always put her family and others first. Betsy had spent decades struggling to lose the same fifteen or twenty pounds she'd been carrying since her first pregnancy. But she shouldn't have been advised to focus on the weight she had to lose. The real threat lay with what she had failed to build. Imaging her brain revealed her future—the pictures I saw looked like those of someone with Alzheimer's. I knew what was in store for her within the next few decades, and it crushed me. I felt that I, along with the mainstream medical community and society, had failed her. To me, she represented dozens of patients I had seen in the same position. Then it hit me.

These people had one thing in common: low muscle mass or some impairment in their muscle. They all lacked the strength to perform certain basic movements (like those listed in chapter 8), and they had low physical tone along with blood markers that indicated unhealthy muscle. Their issue wasn't body fat, I realized; it was a lack of sufficient healthy muscle tissue.

We, in medicine and in society, have long been telling people to lose weight. But by focusing on fat, Betsy, like so many, had failed to get healthy, no matter how hard she tried. I realized that we had gotten the narrative all wrong, and the consequences for countless individual lives would be devastating.

Desperate to repair what I felt was the medical community's biggest failure, Muscle-Centric Medicine® became my mission. I am so grateful for the chance to share with you the groundbreaking science that has the power to revolutionize our pursuit of longevity for extraordinary health at any age.

Do you struggle with constant cravings, low energy, blood-sugar issues, and confusion about what to eat, how to exercise, and why? If so, you are in good company. When I was younger, I obsessed about food and my body weight. I felt hungry all the time and couldn't seem to curb my appetite. I cycled through an array of fad diets, everything from season-determined macrobiotic to all-organic, sprouted, and vegetarian. Back then, before I knew better, my meals were heavily skewed toward an unbalanced diet of carbs often considered healthy, with whole grains like brown rice, barley, millet, oats, and corn. I ate locally grown vegetables, beans and bean products (like tofu, miso, and tempeh), and sea vegetables (like seaweed, nori, and agar). I was chasing after increased energy, health, and athletic performance, but all my careful planning was rooted in misinformation.

I spent hours of each day on food acquisition, obsessing over every tiny detail to get it "right." I avoided parties or brought my own snacks. I exercised for, easily, fourteen hours a week. My focus on food and exercise was unhealthy largely because I thought meeting a baseline of wellness required a diet and training program demanding that much effort. While my intentions were good, this behavior, grounded in my flawed understanding of health, devastated my body and my mind.

After two years, I found myself exhausted and malnourished. Simply put, I had been unintentionally starving myself of the nutrients I needed. Finally, my body's response to growing deficiencies was to start binge eating. Over time, I developed an incredibly disordered relationship with food that stemmed from my inability to regulate hunger. Although I prioritized whole foods, I had completely missed the mark on protein—just like so many other people I've encountered over the years. I was keeping an intense exercise regimen of one hour of cardio plus one hour of weight training daily. Undereating protein left my body starved for extra fuel. All the carbs I ate at that time kept me hungry and at the mercy of constant blood-sugar peaks and crashes. Once I added high-quality, strategically consumed protein to my diet, my suffering began to ease. Finally, I had regained control of my hunger. Proper nutrition helped my body recover from my workouts and supported new growth so I could finally see the results of the effort I'd been putting in. Muscle started forming, and my whole body changed. So did my outlook and eventually my life. Instead of subtracting foods and activities from my life, I started adding.

My struggles with regulating my physiology had left me hungry—not just for food but for understanding too. As I began following discussions about carbohydrates, fats, and proteins, I quickly learned how charged and layered with confusion nutrition can be. Nearly every person I met seemed to have their own beliefs about food science, some personal struggle with nutrition, and an overall fraught long-term relationship with eating that had outlasted any romantic relationship they'd ever been in.

Seeking answers in academia, I noticed that many of my classmates had come to study nutrition out of their own frustrations with food and diet. How had nutrition become such a touchy subject? Why did people eat the foods they ate? Why did some people struggle with weight and food obsession for a lifetime with so little progress?

These initial questions led me to a life spent treating people just like you. Now I'm here to share all I've learned. My greatest desire is to help you find the freedom you've been seeking, just as I did all those years ago.

THE LYON PROTOCOL WORKS

Promoting muscle health is the driving force behind the Lyon Protocol (see more on page 161)—the combination of nutrition and training instructions with operating procedures that will grant you the power to make real, lasting improvements to your body composition and overall health. Muscle-Centric Medicine® and its protein-forward, strength-training-focused lifestyle will change everything. My patients' incredible successes demonstrate just how well these lasting, long-term strategies work.

Within one month of adopting my program and shifting your understanding and your approach from fat-focused to muscle-centric, you will likely gain muscle, lose body fat, and have more energy. Once I teach you how to build a protein-forward nutrition plan, to center your training with a focus on healthy muscle tissue, and to establish mindset guidelines for execution and consistency, you will begin to feel better immediately. And then, farther down the road, you will benefit from improved quality of life and increased longevity.

Time and again, I've observed how quickly my patients' energy levels improve, cravings dissolve, and anxieties ease. Most important, after the Lyon Protocol becomes a part of their routine, they almost immediately develop a sense of inner freedom. My practice has shown me that **once my patients prioritize skeletal muscle as an organ, they gain a whole new sense of wellness.**

My goal is to help you achieve extraordinary health. While maintaining muscle mass demands different strategies for each age group and activity level, your ability to survive and thrive—no matter your age—is directly related to muscle tissue health. Muscle-Centric Medicine®, which recognizes muscle as the organ of longevity, is the future of health. Here's your chance to change your life and rewrite your future.

LOOKING AHEAD

In the coming pages, I will shed light on how we became so blinded to some of the key nutritional realities that have interfered with more widespread health. We will examine the questionable science behind commonly accepted nutritional principles and the deeply misleading "wisdom" that leads so many to poor health outcomes. I will break down the hard-and-fast biological numbers that determine the value of different macro- and micronutrients and will explain what, when, and how to eat and train for maximum health.

Together we'll talk through how you can use your own metrics (including waist circumference, blood triglycerides, high-density lipoproteins, and fasting blood sugar) to take simple, concrete steps to optimize your metabolism, manage your weight, and correct your body composition—energizing your muscles to burn excess calories naturally while protecting your body from inflammation and disease.

YES, THIS BOOK IS FOR YOU

Does any of this sound familiar?

1 Have you followed every program, purchased every diet book, and purposefully and thoughtfully completed every plan, only to find weight loss impossible?

2 Are you highly motivated and creative and a wiz at obtaining information—so much information that you have no idea what to do?

3 Have you been cycling through various juice cleanses, stockpiling enough supplements to open a pharmacy?

4 Did you wake up one day to find yourself wondering, *What happened to my body? What happened to my health?* Did you turn forty and—two kids and a high-stress career later—hardly recognize the person staring back at you in the mirror?

5 Do you suffer from emotional eating? Are you continually backsliding instead of reaching your health goals?

6 Do you struggle to change an unhealthy body composition? ("I'm just big-boned" or "I have a slow metabolism." "Exercise and weight training just don't make a difference for me.")

7 Have you watched your parents age and become immobile and felt helpless to protect them or provide them with a better strategy?

8 Are you fretting about the laundry list of conditions your doctor says you're at risk for, including obesity, osteoporosis, GI problems, poor cognitive function, diabetes, cancer, and even Alzheimer's? Do you see your own future in your parents' predicaments and know, in your gut, that there must be a better way?

9 Are you so busy managing everybody and everything in your life that you can't possibly prioritize your own health needs?

10 Are you settling, convincing yourself you're comfortable where you are, without realizing how much better you could feel?

Whether you're looking to maximize your weight loss and performance or to age well, *Forever Strong* will show you why, when, and what to execute to make real changes in your body and your life.

MINDSET RESET

ADOPTING A GROWTH MINDSET

Before we go any further, I want to lay the groundwork for understanding what I consider the "drivers" of behavior.

Step one is to deconstruct your thinking around health and wellness. Is your mental framework fixed or growth-oriented? The term "growth mindset," popularized by psychologist Dr. Carol Dweck, reminds us of our own mental flexibility and the reality that reaching our full potential takes time and effort. Our beliefs may be powerful, she explains, "but they are just something in your mind, and you can change your mind."[2] Understanding your own mind will help you embrace the new challenges of adopting a muscle-centric lifestyle. A mental framework that welcomes rigor will help you thrive while leveling up both your exercise and nutrition plans. That's because a growth-focused mental framework is the engine that drives progress.

People stuck in a fixed mindset often get caught up in essentialist notions of themselves ("I'm not an athlete"; "I don't like 'health' food"; "I'm gym-phobic"; "I've never been able to stick with a workout plan") and lose sight of their capacity for change. With a growth-mindset approach, on the other hand, we recognize that each of us has the potential to learn new skills and practice new ways of being. Effort is not the end, Dweck insists, but "your means to an end . . . that [is] learning and improving."

Imagine what is possible when we replace:

"I can't do it."

"This is too hard."

"I'm not good at this."
"I'm too old to try new things."

with:
"This may take some time and effort."
"I'm still learning. I'll keep trying."
"I can use a different strategy."
"This will get easier with practice."

Would you let a child struggling to tie her shoe or put on her own jacket throw out a line like "I can't do it" and quit right there? Not likely. Probably, you'd offer some words of encouragement, come up with a "bunny ears" trick for the laces or a lay-it-on-the-floor-first coat-donning strategy, and insist that she keep trying. Why do we sell ourselves short when we know full well how often in this life persistence creates possibility?

Pairing a growth mindset with internal discipline is crucial. I call this integration a growth-focused mental framework. This approach will help you look forward to learning health-improvement skills and enjoy the process—not because it is easy but precisely because it is not. Through challenge comes mental and physical refinement, and that leads to a meaningful life. It's time to recognize that having an "easy" life is a delusion laced with unmet dreams and complacency. If you choose the "easy" path, life will end up being hard; if you choose the hard path, life will wind up easy. I'm here to show you how.

"The ultimate life hack is hard work."
—Dr. Gabrielle Lyon

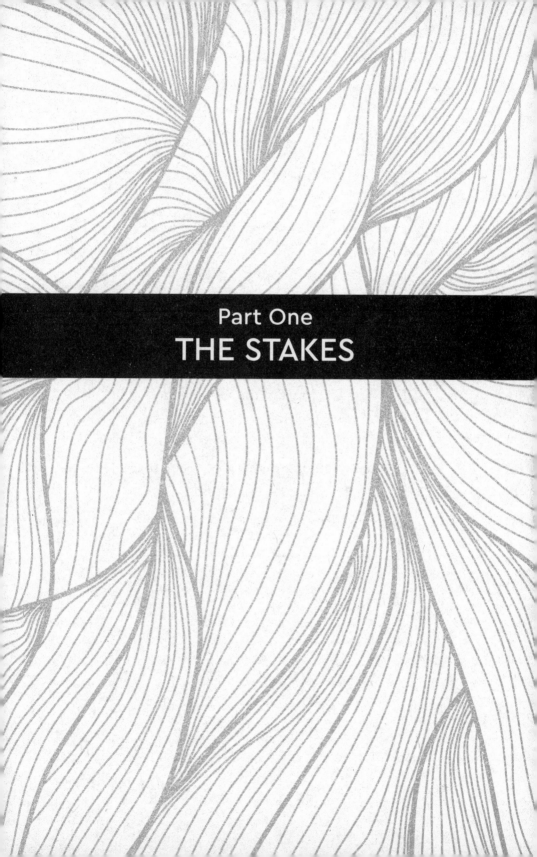

Part One
THE STAKES

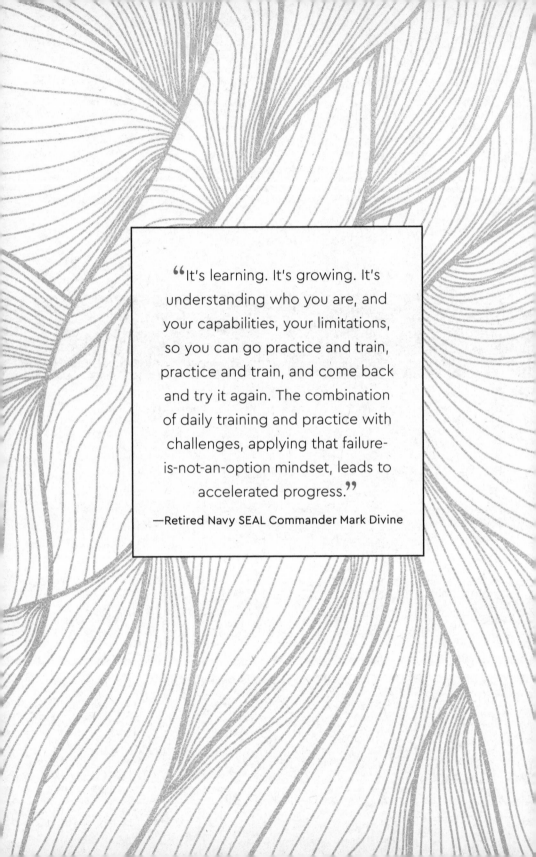

"It's learning. It's growing. It's understanding who you are, and your capabilities, your limitations, so you can go practice and train, practice and train, and come back and try it again. The combination of daily training and practice with challenges, applying that failure-is-not-an-option mindset, leads to accelerated progress."

—Retired Navy SEAL Commander Mark Divine

1.

~~~~~~~~

Shift the Fat-Focused Paradigm

After a lifetime of dieting, my patient Layla decided she'd had enough. A forty-six-year-old chef who suffered from rheumatoid arthritis that left her fatigued and in pain, Layla weighed 317 pounds when she started treatment with me. The medications she needed to keep her immune system in check kept packing on pounds and draining her energy. She was close to giving up.

Layla wasn't alone in her struggle. Obesity is wildly prevalent in the United States. At this point, more than seven out of ten of us are overweight—about 40 percent life-threateningly so! The Centers for Disease Control (CDC) estimates that addressing lifestyle factors such as poor diet, exercise frequency, tobacco smoking, and sleep quality can help to resolve the majority of heart disease, stroke, and type 2 diabetes cases. Additionally, addressing these lifestyle factors reduces risks for specific cancers by up to 40 percent.

And yet, even though we all know we need to eat better and exercise, why is it so hard to implement this change?

Seventy-five percent of Americans don't get the federally recommended weekly minimum of 150 minutes of moderate-intensity exercise (or 75 minutes of vigorous exercise), never mind the two-plus days of full-body strength training recommended by the American College of Sports Medicine (ACSM).[1] Many factors—psychological, physiological, societal, and even religious, as I'll explain in the coming pages—can make it harder for us to get into shape. The trap of feeling exhausted, overwhelmed, and lulled into false ideas about our own abilities to change has prevented us from making the very life changes that build a foundation for long-term health and longevity. If you've reached the point where you think the best thing you can do for yourself at the end of the day is to curl up on the couch and start the binge, dive into an oversized bowl of mac and cheese, pour a large glass of wine, or indulge in a decadent dessert, I'm here to show you another way.

My first goal for Layla was to help her move the needle on the scale. To give her the boost of an early win, step one was to get her moving. She began walking on her lunch break and incorporated three additional ten-minute walks throughout the day. Next, we got Layla started with resistance exercises to assist with quality weight loss that decreased fat tissue without sacrificing muscle. (See more on those in chapter 9.)

Once we got Layla moving, we focused on her nutrition. We anchored her first and last meals with protein, and she eliminated all snacking.

Within seven months, Layla had lost nearly sixty pounds. As exciting, and rare, as that weight loss was, it wasn't even her biggest accomplishment. She was most proud of the health benefits that flowed once her body composition shifted. Her joint pain decreased, allowing her to reduce her arthritis medication. Her blood markers, such as fasting insulin, blood glucose, triglycerides, and hs-CRP, which can gauge risk of coronary artery disease, all improved.

The most inspiring part of her story, though, was realizing that her body *wanted* to get stronger. Shocked by her own success, Layla grew less hungry and more encouraged. She could not believe how easy it was for her to feel so much better. Time and time again, I've witnessed hundreds of my patients transform by following the nutrition and exercise guidelines in the Lyon Protocol. They learn, almost immediately, that **strength is something you can build, inside and out.**

This book is your chance to find clarity in the chaos. The information I'll share on the following pages is meant to help you rise to wellness, on your own terms. Aging is going to happen, no matter what. But the following pages spell out exactly what will arm you against the setbacks to keep your body primed for health that lasts a lifetime.

FORGING A PATH FORWARD

There's no question we need a different approach to health, wellness, and longevity. Beyond the conditions already mentioned, poor muscle health also contributes to Alzheimer's, sarcopenia, osteoporosis, poor cognitive function, polycystic ovary syndrome, fatigue, poor immunity, and even cancer. And yet *all* of us have contended with the confusion and frustration of attempting to navigate the information overload of conflicting health guidelines, particularly when it comes to diet and exercise.

The result is a cycle of mental and physical stress. Contradictory advice leads many of us toward dieting and extended sessions of continuous, cardiovascular exercise that's insufficient to build or protect quality muscle. Regimens that focus on too much aerobic exercise at the expense of resistance training and don't supply sufficient fuel to power muscle growth leave people frustrated and fatigued. If you only do Zumba and skip the weight room, any pounds you lose will include both fat and muscle. Not only does this common, yet misguided, approach sap our motivation and our ability to drive change, but it also depletes the very life-fortifying tissue (aka muscle) that we need to arm ourselves against the forces of aging and disease. Specific, well-timed resistance training (see chapter 9) doesn't just improve your body's composition, but also allows you to perform your daily activities while boosting your metabolic health.

Even my patients who *have* managed to lose weight—which is statistically hard to accomplish and sustain—are also struggling. After months of reducing calories, they wind up shedding pounds but, in the process, losing the wrong kind of weight. This is because traditional weight-loss plans that are focused solely on caloric restriction often lead to unfavorable loss of muscle mass. Then, when the weight piles back on in the form of fat, people wind up even more disheartened than before. Worst of all, each yo-yo cycle through the latest fad diet whittles away the precious muscle tissue that gets harder to gain back with each passing year.

Some of the people I treat have been flooded with plant-based perspectives that have shattered any reasonable nutritional balance and pushed them toward consuming frighteningly high levels of carbs. These folks often wind up struggling with digestive issues and chasing fatigue. (See more on this on page 59.)

The truth is that our society's obsession with fat and lack of focus on skeletal muscle—the internal engine that drives all systems—send people down the wrong path. Over the past decade, I have seen the pain caused by our failed health approaches playing out in the lives of my patients. Like most people, many of them start out with superficial ideas about skeletal muscle—they think about looks, mobility, or functional performance. Strength training can carry stigmas of vanity and "bro science." But muscle does far more essential work than improving appearance or athleticism. Instead, this dynamic tissue, which makes up about 40 percent of a person's mass, is the keystone organ of health. Healthy muscle is imperative to a body's function. That's why, if you want to change your body—inside and out—repairing damaged muscle and building new lean muscle mass form the critical first step.

THE LIFE-CHANGING POWER OF SKELETAL MUSCLE

Skeletal muscle (the muscle that moves bones to control our locomotion) not only constructs our physical architecture but also impacts our physiological infrastructure. A grossly underestimated resource, muscle burns fat, drives metabolism, protects against disease, and so much more.

Nearly immediate improvements (measurable within two weeks) brought about by increasing muscle health include **better blood-sugar regulation, hunger control, and increased mobility.**

Longer-term benefits include **a stronger body and stronger bones, an improved blood profile including lower triglycerides, metabolism protection, increased survivability against nearly every disease, and a better mood.**

Muscle-Centric Medicine® harnesses this powerful system to **heal disease, build better body composition, boost energy, increase mobility, and combat the conditions associated with aging.**

Consider skeletal muscle as your body armor and the Lyon Protocol as your battle plan. *Forever Strong* will show you what to do and how to train your mind to *get the job done.* Nurtured through nutrition, lifestyle, and proper exercise, healthy muscle tissue brings endless health benefits, ultimately holding the key to aging *the way you want to* rather than the ways society convinces you to accept. The better your habits, the more dialed-in your execution, the more you will be able to attain excellence in this personal sphere. Treat your muscles right, and the results will astound you. I'm here to show you how.

ALL ABOUT MUSCLE: THE ORGAN OF LONGEVITY

Building muscle is the most important safeguard for health because it is the bodily system that will allow us to live our longest, most capable, fulfilling life.

The key is metabolic health. By increasing your healthy muscle mass, you not only change your body's physical structure but also direct how your body uses both food and energy. Through training, you increase the density of muscle mitochondria—the primary energy-producing units within almost every cell of the body. This allows your body to use nutrients, such as carbohydrates and fats, and convert them into energy that can be used to power everyday activities. Training also boosts your immune function via peptides—small molecules composed of amino acids—released during muscle contraction. Key peptides can send signals in the body that help fight off germs and reduce inflammation.

On the flip side, unhealthy muscle is not only weaker but also less effective as a metabolic sink. In essence, building muscle creates something like body armor that protects you in *all* domains of health. What you do and how you live—in particular, what you eat and how you exercise—dramatically affect this organ system both immediately and over the long term. Through specific, targeted behaviors, you can literally change your destiny by empowering your muscle to run the body's energy-processing and chemical-messaging system in healthy ways.

BACK TO LIFE SCIENCE CLASS
(BUT I PROMISE IT WILL BE BRIEF)

Let me take a minute now to break down for you the basics of cellular function and explain the way muscles utilize the nutrients provided through food. First, it helps to understand that the primary sugar you obtain from food is glucose—a vital nutrient that's essential for proper brain, heart, and digestive function, as well as maintaining healthy vision and skin. Research shows that glucose—not fat or protein—is the primary determinant of muscle metabolic fuel preferences.[2] The body prioritizes burning and storing glucose, over fat and protein, because if blood sugar levels remain too high for too long, glucose becomes toxic. (*Note: Everything* can be toxic to the body at some amount; it just depends on the dose. One can even overdose on water!) Indeed, poor glucose clearance, as is seen in insulin resistance and diabetes, damages the tissues of the body.

Our bodies use multiple mechanisms to dispose of the excess glucose we've ingested within a maximum of two hours. We can measure the success of this process through an oral glucose tolerance test, which reveals how much time it takes our bodies to clear this sugar from the circulation. The less time it takes, the more insulin sensitive or glucose tolerant one is said to be.

I'll explain all of this in greater detail a little later, but one key health strategy I'll be teaching you is how to mitigate glucose responses by properly dosing your carbohydrates at each meal. I'll explain how detrimental reaching for carb-heavy snacks can be for both your weight-loss and metabolic-health optimization goals. Metabolic dysfunction is the leading driver of most of the diseases we face as a society. It makes for unhealthy muscle, infiltrated with fat, much like a marbled steak. This can lead to chronic fatigue, loss of strength, and insulin resistance, as well as the limitation of daily activities.

To combat these effects, we need to grow our muscles and turn them into mitochondria-manufacturing plants. Declines in muscle mass and mitochondria diminish the body's capacity to store and burn glucose, resulting in an overburdened insulin system that's working overtime to try to find places to dispose of this nutrient. The most important thing to understand right now is that **it is absolutely possible to optimize or restore proper metabolic function by building and maintaining healthy muscle.**

In addition to facilitating glucose disposal, muscle tissue also serves as one of the largest sites of fatty acid oxidation. Fatty acids can be categorized into four main groups: saturated, monounsaturated, polyunsaturated, and trans fatty acids. At rest, muscle burns fatty acids as its primary energy source.

Currently, forty million Americans are prescribed statins to lower their LDL cholesterol caused by metabolic dysfunction, while receiving virtually no guidance on optimizing metabolic health by improving muscle quality and quantity. The more healthy muscle tissue you have to process fat and glucose, the more metabolically healthy you will be, and the less you will need to rely on pharmacological interventions.

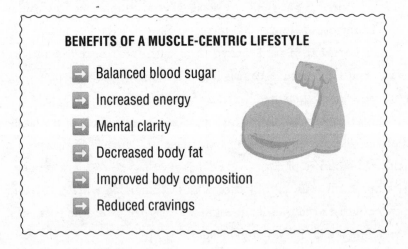

BENEFITS OF A MUSCLE-CENTRIC LIFESTYLE

→ Balanced blood sugar

→ Increased energy

→ Mental clarity

→ Decreased body fat

→ Improved body composition

→ Reduced cravings

Skeletal muscle also acts as an amino-acid reservoir, keeping these fundamental nutrients flowing in your body in the absence of food. This is the metabolic duty of muscle. If you become sick or injured, the body will pull amino acids from your available muscle tissue to repair and protect itself. Multiple studies have shown that the healthier your muscles, the greater your survivability when things go wrong. In fact, a person's ability to survive cachexia, a wasting disease often associated with cancer, is directly related to total muscle mass.

THE METABOLIC POWER OF MUSCLE

By highlighting muscle as your target for better health, you can create positive momentum focused on *what you have to gain* rather than *what you need to lose*. Given the power of muscle to help stave off diseases commonly attributed to aging, we should be thinking of muscle as a new health end point.

A typical doctor's visit includes measuring vital signs such as blood pressure, pulse, and weight. But for a more accurate picture of overall health, your doctor should also be measuring your muscle mass at each annual visit, with a strength assessment and other tests. This would allow immediate feedback about the trending direction of your muscle condition, which ultimately determines so much about your overall health. Until the medical system steps up to the challenge, it's crucial that you take charge of your own longevity.

Muscle health has two major components: (1) physical and (2) metabolic. The physical involves strength and mass, while the metabolic affects insulin sensitivity, glucose regulation, fatty-acid oxidation, and mitochondria health. Often called the powerhouses of a cell, mitochondria play a critical role in converting the food we eat into energy our cells can use. Their health determines the wellness of our tissue and organs, while their dysfunction can cause life-threatening conditions.

To understand how muscle helps drive metabolism and why its effect is so important, it helps to grasp three core concepts:

1 Glucose becomes toxic to the body when too much remains in the bloodstream for too long, that is, more than two hours. (We call this disease state diabetes.)

2 Insulin is the body's main mechanism for removing glucose from the bloodstream.

3 A root cause of obesity and related diseases (including type 2 diabetes, hypertension, cardiovascular disease, and impaired fertility, among other conditions) is decreased insulin sensitivity, also known as insulin resistance.

Now, here's where exercise comes in. **Muscle contraction during both aerobic and resistance training stimulates the uptake of glucose *without* any need for insulin's assistance.** This insulin-independent uptake offers an additional effective mechanism for removing excess glucose from the blood. And check out this bonus: in response to resistance training, specifically, your body reaps the benefits of contraction-driven glucose uptake **for up to two days after your workout** because exercise improves insulin-stimulated glucose uptake. During the post-workout window, the increased density of glucose transporters present in muscle cell membranes continue their work of getting rid of excess blood glucose, still with less insulin required. Here's another benefit: the glucose that gets stored in your muscle tissue as glycogen fuels both short, intense exercise and longer endurance training. In other words, with proper nutrition, the glycogen resynthesized after your workout **gives you back the energy you need to keep training.** As you can see, this system works on a feedback loop. Exercise not only helps manage proper blood-sugar and insulin levels, but it also primes the muscle. As exercise burns glycogen (glucose) it leaves the post-exercise muscle tissue primed for glucose uptake. Proper nutritional refueling then replenishes glycogen stores, helping your body meet its ongoing training needs, thereby powering this healthy energy cycle over the long haul. Understanding the interplay of these dynamics offers a lifelong solution.[3]

Now let's look at what happens in the opposite scenario, where the muscle is not sufficiently worked, hindering all the positive effects exercise can have on the whole system.

DROP THE BAGGAGE

Think of muscle as a suitcase. When you continue to eat the wrong foods in the wrong quantities, you overstuff your suitcase until the excess contents spill out. In this case, what spills out is glucose, fatty acids, or amino acids, and all that substrate overflows back into the bloodstream. Somehow the body must dispose of all those extras. That's when initial disease processes begin. Whether the trouble starts as obesity, diabetes, or other conditions, the underlying pathology remains the same. When muscle, your main metabolic organ, gets flooded and overwhelmed, you gain fat. This fat goes on to create low-grade inflammation. When you have unhealthy muscle, poor diet choices can create postprandial inflammation every time you eat, hurting muscle's metabolic regulation and causing a whole host of other problems.[4]

Skeletal muscle health issues often begin early in life. When we are young and seem healthy enough, we think we can get away with less-than-optimal choices—even being sedentary—because we don't see a change in clothing size. In reality, **there is no such thing as "healthy" inactive**. What we commonly think of as diseases of aging are really diseases of impaired muscle.

The information I'm providing here about the function of muscle as an organ upends completely the mainstream understanding of the relationships between food, exercise, fat, and muscle. Grasping these interactions will arm you with all you need to reprioritize muscle health in the life decisions you make. **Optimizing your muscle will optimize your life.**

FIVE WAYS TO MAKE MUSCLE MAGIC

❶ Every hour, complete 10 to 20 air squats.

❷ Stand at your desk.

❸ Get your heart rate up with a brisk walk to the bathroom or water fountain 10 times a day.

❹ Bring a resistance band to your office to get in a quick 10-rep set of bicep curls between tasks.

❺ Wear a lightly weighted vest to work to add in just a little more resistance.

BREAKING IT DOWN: INSULIN RESISTANCE

Insulin is a peptide hormone released from the pancreas to move glucose into cells. Too little insulin is deadly. Too much is also deadly. When insulin resistance leads the body to require more insulin, this creates a state that drives metabolic disease and derangement in blood lipids. A pivotal paper from Kitt Petersen demonstrated that insulin resistance in skeletal muscle, due to challenges with muscle glycogen synthesis (think of that overstuffed suitcase), can promote elevated levels of triglycerides (TG) and low-density lipoprotein (LDL) cholesterol along with low levels of high-density lipoprotein (HDL) cholesterol.[5]

The insulin resistance experienced by these individuals was *independent of changes in intra-abdominal obesity.* See what I'm getting at here? If insulin resistance shows up without extra abdominal fat appearing, fat tissue and obesity may not play a primary role in causing insulin resistance in the early stages of the metabolic syndrome!

While the liver is another critical organ in this story, the most functional way to disrupt this unhealthy progression is through building skeletal muscle. Why? Because the last time I checked, it's not possible to exercise your liver. Further, the sheer mass of muscle makes it a more effective tissue to target.

The science clearly shows that skeletal muscle is an area of initial insult that leads to insulin resistance in other areas of the body, resulting in type 2 diabetes. The authors of one of my favorite papers express this succinctly in their title, "Skeletal Muscle Insulin Resistance Is the Primary Defect in Type 2 Diabetes." [6] A decade or more before beta-cell failure in the pancreas (the linchpin of diabetes) results in elevated fasting blood-sugar levels, insulin resistance can already be detected within skeletal muscle.

Therefore, if you want to correct for the body's insulin resistance, it makes sense to focus on the largest primary site of this resistance in the body. That way, you are hitting the highest-value target. Achieving—and maintaining—proper insulin regulation requires, first, emptying the proverbial tank and, second, keeping skeletal muscle healthy.

MUSCLE AS A BLOOD-SUGAR-STABILIZING ORGAN

Not only does muscle help with preventing high blood-glucose levels, but it also helps prevent levels from dropping too low. In the absence of dietary carbohydrates, amino acids released by muscle can be used to synthesize glucose in the liver, which directly supports blood-glucose levels. This mechanism allows muscle to assist in blood-sugar stabilization.

By adjusting your protein intake and prioritizing training to meet your metabolic goals, you can mitigate the effects of aging, such as the decline of the natural steroids (i.e., anabolic hormones) like testosterone that stimulate muscle protein synthesis and muscle growth while protecting against insulin resistance. Increasing protein intake also protects your body's ability to regenerate tissue while also stimulating the nutrient-sensing capacity of muscle tissue, allowing it to use dietary protein most efficiently. All these factors support your efforts to hold on to muscle. Let's dive a little deeper into the nutrient-sensing capacity I just mentioned. It turns out muscle is remarkably malleable and responsive. We've already discussed how skeletal muscle reacts biochemically to contractile forces (i.e., exercise) in beneficial ways. It also responds directly to nutrition like no other organ. Muscle can sense the protein you eat and proceed with stimulating growth of new tissue based on the availability of sufficient and appropriate amino acids. Amino acids are the building blocks of proteins—the biomolecules that establish the physical structure of the body and facilitate all of the metabolic reactions required for life.

Don't worry! I'll explain all of this in greater detail in chapter 5, feeding you all the facts, figures, and equations to help you establish the nutrient balance that your body needs based on your current situation and your future goals.

METABOLISM: SOLVING MYSTERIES
AND MISCONCEPTIONS

OK, are you ready to have your mind blown?

You might have heard that muscle plays the biggest role in using calories and elevating our metabolism while we're at rest. But don't be fooled. Although muscle does play a huge role in moving the metabolism needle, the reason is not what you might think.

Here's what you'll hear at the gym: Every 10 kg difference in lean mass translates to a difference in energy expenditure of approximately 100 kcal per day. This means that **every hard-earned pound of muscle burns only about 10 calories at rest.** Now, most people right about now are thinking, *Wait a second! All that effort just to burn a measly 10 extra calories?* The fact is that the calories you burn from simply having muscle is *not* the primary effect, despite how often this information is repeated.

We know that exercise blazes through calories, but the metabolic power is this: well-trained muscle tissue is more efficient and effective at utilizing calories. So healthy muscle tissue *does* increase your metabolism but in a different way from how you likely understood it previously. Muscle boosts metabolism by using energy for protein turnover. **The more healthy muscle you have, the greater ability your body has to stay in homeostasis or balance.**

You've doubtless heard that "calories in versus calories out" creates weight loss or gain. This metric is used to describe the major elements determining our energy expenditure, with the goal of reaching exceptional health and wellness goals. But from a muscle-centric perspective, we must reconsider the very foundation of this equation, incorporating effects from the laws of thermodynamics. Here you'll see that even this simple equation, rooted in the binary thinking we've used for decades, has blinded us to other important pieces of the puzzle.

The troubles caused by visceral obesity and the effects of aging on muscle strength are well established.[7] To debunk a pervasive myth about obesity, excess fat gets stored not just in adipose tissue but in other tissues as well—including muscle. This spells bad news in terms of actual strength (peak muscle force generation) and metabolic health, along with a multitude of other unwelcome outcomes. Beyond the devastating impairments of mobility and metabolism, intramuscular adipose tissue (IMAT) is a significant predictor of conditions such as stroke, spinal-cord injury, diabetes, and chronic obstructive pulmonary disease (COPD).

The fates I've just outlined aren't pretty, but here's the good news. We all have within us powerful tools for improving our muscle health. You can reverse some, if not all, of the damage to your muscle. With adequate stimulus from diet and exercise, you can move the needle from sarcopenic to strong, at any age.

MYOKINE MAGIC

In the same way that your thyroid releases specific hormones that regulate your weight, energy levels, and internal temperature, muscle tissue releases small signaling proteins known as myokines that act both locally and system-wide. Skeletal muscle's ability to release these circulating hormone-like proteins **establishes muscle tissue as an endocrine organ**. In plain English, that means skeletal muscle releases substances that travel in the bloodstream and influence other cells to help regulate multiple body functions, far beyond simple locomotion. Myokines released in response to muscle contractions during exercise play a significant role in energy utilization. These proteins, which help regulate metabolism in all body tissues, also exert specific, health-boosting, anti-inflammatory effects on different tissues, while improving immune function and metabolism.[8]

If you haven't heard about the role of muscle as an endocrine organ before, that's because this relatively new concept is still foreign to many of us, including many medical professionals. Pioneering research established muscle contraction's power to influence metabolism through the stimulation, production, and release of disease-fighting cytokines.

At the same time, it opened a whole new paradigm: instituting skeletal muscle as an endocrine organ—in fact, the largest organ system in the human body.[9] It is, perhaps, the most important organ system for combating our current health crisis, regaining exceptional health, and maximizing physical performance.

Learning about these powerful molecules dramatically transformed my own thinking about food and exercise by impressing upon me the critical function of muscle. This research showed me how important it is to eat in a way that allows the body to store less fat while using exercise as a potent tool to elicit metabolic changes. Your quality of life correlates directly with your muscle health. If your muscles are healthy, you live better.

Beyond the benefits already mentioned, new science reveals yet another major health boost provided by resistance training: increased production and release of myokines. Myokines are a collection of small proteins and peptides secreted into the bloodstream during skeletal-muscle contraction. Because they act as chemical signals that produce downstream metabolic and hormonal changes, myokines help your body metabolize glucose from your bloodstream *without* the use of insulin. This effect benefits everyone, but it can offer significant metabolic correction for insulin-resistant individuals. Actively working and taxing your muscle tissue will not only help regulate your hormones but will also make you better able to regulate your blood sugar and improve your body composition.

Myokines even improve your sense of well-being and capacity to learn. Studies have shown that working out increases blood flow to the brain, promoting the development of new brain cells while helping to clear out toxins.[10] During exercise, muscle releases two myokines called cathepsin B and irisin, which can enter the circulation and cross the blood-brain barrier, where they stimulate the production of brain-derived neurotrophic factor (BDNF). This uptick in BDNF boosts neurogenesis, or the formation of new neurons, facilitating learning and memory.[11] Higher levels of BDNF correlate with decreased incidence of mood disorders, while aerobic-exercise-induced increases in BDNF are associated with increased volume in the hippocampus—the region of the brain that facilitates learning, memory, and spatial awareness.[12]

The takeaway is this: you'd be shocked to learn just how much muscle you still have the capacity to build—even if you're struggling with a long-term illness or feel like you've missed the boat on getting healthy—and how big a role it will play in saving your life. Read more to learn how!

If you are a health coach or personal trainer who wants to implement Muscle-Centric Medicine® to help your clients achieve long-term results, visit www.drgabrielleyon.com to learn more about my courses!

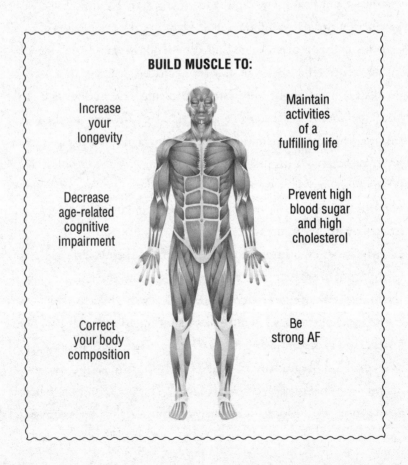

BUILD MUSCLE TO:

Increase your longevity

Maintain activities of a fulfilling life

Decrease age-related cognitive impairment

Prevent high blood sugar and high cholesterol

Correct your body composition

Be strong AF

MINDSET RESET

HARNESS YOUR THOUGHTS

What makes elite military operators, high-performing CEOs, and other hugely successful individuals so different from others? Mental framework. They don't get derailed by any mental chatter that moves them off the mark. The key is to train your mind to become an asset rather than a liability. My longtime mentor and friend former commander Mark Divine taught me that we can learn to neutralize negative self-talk and harness our own thinking patterns.

In my clinical practice, I work with anyone who's ready to level up in their lives, whether they're an athlete, an executive, a parent, a Navy SEAL, or some combination. The thing that brings them into my office is the promise of wellness. But that's just the entry point for the even more meaningful internal restructuring that we cultivate together. Medicine is the modality I use to give people a more victorious life. I tell all my patients, the first muscle you need to work on is between your ears. The same goes for you, dear reader. In building out an organizational framework to guide you on your path toward real and lasting results, I'll leverage all the experience I have with setting up my patients for success.

Achieving your wellness goals depends on two core factors: **knowing WHAT to do**, that is, absorbing the evidence-based guidance I'm sharing about diet, exercise, and other lifestyle interventions, and **knowing HOW to do it**. By HOW, I do not just mean the technical steps of planning a meal or programming a workout (although I provide lots of good detail on both those subjects in chapter 7 and chapter 9, as well as on my YouTube channel). What I'm referring to here is harnessing the mental framework necessary, in all its layers, to get the job done.

The job at hand is taking 100 percent control of, and responsibility for, your own well-being. The only thing we can control is our thoughts, so let's start there. That work begins with bringing to awareness the unconscious mental factors operating in the background.

The HOW involves governing your own mental landscape. By learning to navigate your own acrobatic mind, you can identify strengths and weaknesses, navigate pitfalls, and seize control of internal logistics. This approach is concerned not with goal setting but rather with standard setting that will help you face your hidden fears and release the handcuffs preventing you from living your best life. We'll take this same top-down approach with both your nutritional and physical training. Your increasing mental strength will help shape your growing physical strength and vice versa. Together, they build grit and resilience.

Consider these scenarios: Do you usually feel positive about yourself but turn to self-destructive behaviors after a tense business meeting or a fight with your spouse? Do you say, "I deserve this cake" or "I just need a drink after such a long day"? Maybe these patterns lead you to gain extra weight. Maybe you wind up convinced that *you* are the failure, rather than realizing it's your plan that needs tweaking. Instead of playing the shame-and-blame game, consider what you can learn from the experience. Notice the pitfalls. Where are the holes in your safety net? What guardrails can you erect for the next time?

2.

~~~~~~~~~

Thwart Disease

N o matter how many times you've gained and lost the same amount of weight, **you can repair your metabolism and your muscle tissue**. Even muscle that's already infiltrated with fat? YES! The Lyon Protocol, which I break down on page 161, allows you to both improve the health of your existing muscle and build more.

When we evaluate our health, many of us focus on the immediate, day-to-day, hour-to-hour sensory experiences of wellness. But we rarely take the time to connect these symptoms to the long-term repercussions they represent. Consider these examples: fatigue, memory, mood, and blood-sugar regulation. Know what they all have in common? These are just a few of the key perceptible health benchmarks managed by muscle tissue.

Typically speaking, the Western medical system skews its emphasis toward what's making us sick while overlooking prevention. This tendency leads many doctors to focus on fat and glucose while disregarding the skeletal muscle that could correct the imbalance. Instead of stopping the spin cycle of illness, we're sent chasing our tails. To combat this oversight and highlight the critical role of muscle in long-term health, **I propose that muscle mass be considered as an end-point goal of its own—a biomarker for overall health.**[1]

THE REAL FOUNTAIN OF YOUTH

My goal is nothing short of upending modern medicine with a re-focus on muscle as the fountain of youth. In real life, it's neither a fantastical elixir nor a miraculous curative. But muscle can still be a magic pill for transforming health outcomes. And fortunately, muscle also happens to be **the only organ over which we can voluntarily exert control**. Accepting this minor miracle will empower you to shift into execution mode to improve your health, starting now.

Here's a maxim to keep you motivated: **the higher your healthy muscle mass, the greater your protection against all-cause mortality and morbidity.**

Are you able to perform your daily activities? Do you experience pain throughout the day? Do you feel healthy? Do you have the energy to do the things you love? These are the key factors to consider as you evaluate your current health and gear up for making improvements. Preventing and managing the following common conditions are the most potent ways of feeling strong and staying young.

SARCOPENIA

Each of us is aging every day, and long before we might see the effects on the outside, our bodies are changing out of view. If we don't work hard to maintain muscle, we find ourselves at a strong risk for sarcopenia—the progressive decline in muscle mass due to aging that results in a decreased functional capacity of the muscle tissue.[2]

We have all seen sarcopenia in action. Maybe you've watched older relatives seem to shrink from year to year as they struggle to sort through wave after wave of conflicting health information or simply give up altogether.

Maybe you've noticed your own muscle wasting after having a cast removed, leaving a small, pale, weak limb that's a fraction of the size it was when the cast went on. After I broke my scapula, my arm was immobilized in a sling for weeks. When I was finally able to use my arm again, I could hardly believe how much strength and size I'd lost. In each of these instances, we can see what happens when the body isn't able to properly repair and replace tissues.

While commonly associated with frailty in "old age," sarcopenia can begin in your thirties, just like dementia and heart disease. Understanding and addressing the challenges that result from inactivity and suboptimal protein consumption is vital to overcoming fat gain and muscle loss in later life.

Which does more damage, losing muscle or gaining fat? The answer is losing muscle. A study of elderly men comparing obesity with sarcopenia found that compared with high fat mass, low muscle mass both increased risk of injury and had a greater negative impact on performance. Supporting a muscle-centric perspective on longevity, these findings demonstrate the importance of building muscle to protect you as you age.[3] Losing muscle quality means you lose the metabolic advantages of muscle, specifically power, strength, and mitochondria. Importantly, these disadvantages can occur when muscle tissue is lost at *any* age.

By understanding muscle as the key to longevity and taking action to rebalance the effects of losing and gaining muscle, you can slow the process of aging. As you get older, the body's breakdown of muscle (catabolism) proceeds at an accelerated rate. Left unchecked, the body goes into a state of constant decline. By shifting the balance to a more favorable process of building muscle (anabolism), you protect yourself from catabolism for as long as possible. This will help fend off the negative consequences of the higher states of inflammation, as happens when obesity sets in, that push your metabolic balance to a state where gaining and keeping healthy muscle are harder.

People with obesity and low-grade inflammation have difficulty gaining muscle, yet that's precisely what they need to improve and sustain their health. The reasons are multifold. First, chronic inflammation causes a blunted response to exercise, and muscle damaged by fat and sedentary behavior does not sense nutrients as robustly, respond as effectively to exercise, or recover properly after a workout. Decreased muscle responsiveness makes it harder to get back to a state of balance that can help protect against Alzheimer's disease, cardiovascular disease, and hypertension, among other conditions. Still, taking strategic action can help people overcome obesity's effects.

It's not too late to make the diet and exercise changes (*hint:* following the Lyon Protocol) that can melt away that muscle marbling and get you back on track to health.

People with less muscle mass have lower rates of survival from nearly all diseases. During times of infection, physical trauma, and cancer, the human body requires a significant influx of amino acids. The body sources these from its own amino acid reservoirs: muscle tissue. The more high-quality muscle tissue you have to draw from, the longer you can survive.

Let's consider an extreme case. As a medical student, I spent time studying burn reconstruction. For normal burn healing (depending on wound size), patients required, easily, three times the protein recommended by the USDA.[4] This protein intake was necessary to provide the materials for the protein synthesis that helps to rebuild and structure new tissue. During times of accelerated healing, the amino acid requirements of most tissues, including liver cells and immune cells (which rely heavily on the amino acid glutamine), increase significantly.

Burn-unit healing might seem like a dramatic example, but the fact is our bodies are regularly working to heal while coping with various states of stress. This example highlights our increased need for protein for physical healing of all sorts. Providing adequate protein and associated vitamins and minerals allows for more rapid recovery while sparing precious muscle tissue.

IMMUNE SYSTEM BASICS

The immune system comprises two distinct branches: innate immunity and adaptive immunity. The innate immune system encompasses the body's first line of defenses against a wide array of invaders and includes immune barriers (i.e., skin, mucosa), stomach acid, and immune cells that target pathogens for destruction nonspecifically. Conversely, the adaptive immune system generates unique responses to specific pathogens and then remembers these responses for future encounters.

Cells and organs team up to protect the body. Phagocytes—a class of white blood cells that includes bacteria-fighting neutrophils—act like a Pac-Man chomping up invading organisms. Lymphocytes help the body remember the invaders and facilitate their destruction upon future encounters. I think of B lymphocytes as the body's military intelligence system. Like the CIA, B lymphocytes locate their targets and send out defenses. Like the soldiers sent in to destroy counterforces, defense-system T lymphocytes (or T cells) are the cells that lock onto and disable invaders.

The immune system relies on B lymphocytes to locate and eliminate foreign substances (antigens). Alerted by the body, the immune system prompts B lymphocytes to make antibodies (also called immunoglobulins). These proteins lock onto specific antigens, defusing their power. After they're made, antibodies usually stay in our system to help us fight future battles against invaders. What does all this have to do with muscle? Hold tight and you'll see.

How Muscle Fuels the Immune System

Many studies have shown the importance of regular exercise and physical activity for increasing the body's ability to fight infections over the long haul. This is important to consider not only in response to a novel virus pandemic, for example, but also as a strategy for fighting other established diseases. Because we have the power to voluntarily control our skeletal muscle, resistance training offers an important tool for immune-system enhancement.

The myokines released by your skeletal muscle impact both the innate and adaptive branches of your immune system. In particular, two myokines secreted in response to exercise, IL-6 and IL-15, have been shown to significantly affect immunity. Muscle tissue releases IL-6 during steady-state aerobic training and releases IL-15 largely during resistance training and somewhat from cardio.[5] While muscle's effects on the immune system typically go unseen, we can use lab testing to sneak a glimpse of these processes at work. We are looking into ways to analyze blood markers to gauge the effectiveness of skeletal muscle as an organ system. Results from specific blood panels not only reveal some aspects of overall muscle health but also can be used, along with other health biomarkers, to direct and quantify the specific impacts of exercise on our immune function.[6]

New research reinforces this new model of looking at exercise in a dose-response manner. We've long known that an elevated total white blood cell (WBC) count is associated with an increased risk of coronary heart disease and death and that aerobic exercise is associated with lower total WBC counts. Until recently, however, no studies had examined what impact a specific *amount*, or *dose*, of aerobic exercise would have on these counts. In the DREW study, sedentary, overweight/obese postmenopausal women were enrolled in an aerobic training program for six months. The women were split into three groups with differing weekly exercise requirements. One group was instructed to burn 2 kcal/lb body weight weekly during exercise, the second burned 4 kcal/lb body weight weekly, and the third burned 8 kcal/lb body weight weekly. Strikingly, the results of this study revealed a dose-dependent reduction in WBC counts; the women who burned the most calories during exercise received the largest benefits. This evidence builds upon findings from a 2012 randomized trial revealing how increased physical activity significantly reduces risk of cardiovascular disease morbidity, especially in women with systemic low-grade inflammation.[7]

Exercise and Autoimmune Diseases

According to the National Institutes of Health (NIH), 25 million Americans are affected by more than eighty autoimmune diseases.[8] These illnesses are characterized by autoimmune malfunction, in which the body begins to attack its own tissues, and are triggered by environmental toxins, infections, and genetic factors. Diagnoses such as rheumatoid arthritis and lupus, among others, deeply affect people's lives. In many cases, common clinical features that have physical and mental implications on wellness, such as pain, chronic fatigue, and depression, are both caused and compounded by lack of physical activity. Collectively, these affect up to 23.5 million people in the US, and studies suggest these numbers are rising.

A quick Google search of treatments for autoimmune diseases results in a lengthy list of prescription medications and surgical options. The current standard of care in medical treatment involves drugs that suppress the immune system: steroids and biologics. The mainstays of treatment—glucocorticoids and immunosuppressive drugs—typically provide only short-term relief and often come with significant side effects, including damage to skeletal muscle, which is the very organ with the capacity to help regulate these diseases. Using these drugs over the long term has been associated with bone and muscle mass wasting as well as cardiovascular dysfunction—the exact opposite of the long, healthy life we're working toward here! Moreover, these medications may not effectively hamper the progression of disabilities because they can destroy the very tissues that offer protection.

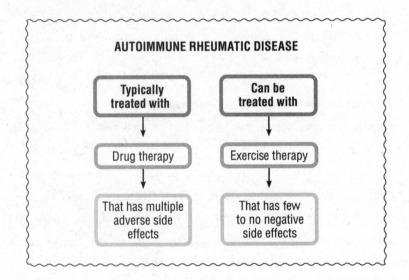

While some people may need these medications, depending on symptom severity, a vast majority are able to significantly improve their quality of life by changing the basics:

- getting outdoors for a walk,
- beginning weight training, and
- simply starting to move your body can help with relieving pain and stiffness.

The science is clear that autoimmune diseases are more prevalent among people who don't exercise. Studies also show that healthy muscle and physical activity could augment treatment by elevating regulatory T cells and inducing an anti-inflammatory response that helps regulate immune health.[9] Keep in mind that one of the driving forces of these diseases is the sustained inflammation that keeps the body's defenses on constant high alert.

Research clearly shows that skeletal muscle plays a role in regulating a healthy immune system. In my practice, nearly 100 percent of my patients with these diseases feel tremendously better using exercise versus medications. Absolutely, talk to your doctor if you're experiencing severe symptoms. But also begin an exercise routine and notice the positive benefits for your body.

Overall, muscle serves as a kind of biological clock, switching on pathology when the tissue is unhealthy or allowing for physiological solutions when muscle quality is maintained. In other words, **the condition of your muscle tissue can heighten disease processes or correct metabolism as well as the underlying disease.** Don't you want to start building before disease sets in?

CANCER

Cancer is a complex set of disease processes that even the best and brightest minds don't yet completely understand. Risks both known and unknown leave us exposed to malignancy. Because we all experience some degree of DNA damage, all our bodies are susceptible to cancers of various types. Further complicating matters are the false risk associations between some foods and cancers that muddy the waters with dangerous myths. We'll discuss these dietary factors a little later. For now, I want to explain the basic mechanisms of cancer to build a baseline understanding so we can examine critically the information that's out there in the world.

Cancer impacts tens of millions of people a year.[10] By 2040, the global cancer burden will grow to 27.5 million new cases and 16.3 million deaths, according to American Cancer Society predictions. Malignancy begins with an initiation phase resulting from a genetic alteration caused by exposures such as smoking, sun, alcohol, and others that drive oncogenic—that is, tumor-producing—effects. We know that cancer and obesity are linked and that body fat is a modifiable risk factor. One reason is the DNA damage that low-grade inflammation from excess adipose tissue causes over time. Other factors include the varied metabolic abnormalities associated with a high percentage of visceral fat tissue. The Western diet, in particular, is strongly linked to liver, pancreatic, and kidney cancers (to name a few).

We know that overweight and obese individuals are more likely than healthy-weight individuals to have conditions or disorders linked to chronic local inflammation.[11] One remedy for this risk factor is building, maintaining, and optimizing for healthy muscle. Obesity is strongly linked to increased risk of thirteen different cancers; here are just a handful.

■ **Endometrial cancer:** Healthy-weight women are significantly less likely than obese and overweight women to develop endometrial cancer (cancer of the lining of the uterus). The risk of endometrial cancer increases with weight gain in adulthood.[12]

- **Esophageal adenocarcinoma:** Healthy-weight people are two times less likely than those who are overweight or obese to develop a type of esophageal cancer called esophageal adenocarcinoma, while people who are extremely obese are more than four times more likely.[13]

- **Gastric cardia cancer:** Overweight and obese individuals have an approximately two times greater risk for gastric cardia cancer compared with healthy-weight people.[14]

- **Pancreatic cancer:** Healthy-weight people are about 1.5 times less likely to develop pancreatic cancer than people who are overweight or obese.[15]

- **Colorectal cancer:** A higher body mass index (BMI) is associated with increased risks of colon and rectal cancers in both men and women, with larger increases in men.[16]

- **Gallbladder cancer:** Compared with healthy-weight people, those who are overweight or obese have an increased risk of gallbladder cancer, with a 5 percent increased risk for every five BMI units.[17] This risk increase is slightly greater in women than in men.

- **Breast cancer:** Many studies have shown that in postmenopausal women, a higher BMI is associated with a modest increase in risk of breast cancer. For example, a five-unit increase in BMI is associated with a 12 percent increase in risk.[18] Healthy-weight postmenopausal women have a 20 to 40 percent decreased risk of developing estrogen-receptor-positive breast cancer compared with those who are obese.[19]

- **Ovarian cancer:** Higher BMI is associated with a slight increase in the risk of ovarian cancer, particularly in women who have never used menopausal hormone therapy.[20]

Wondering what you're supposed to do with all these grim statistics? My goal is not to depress you but to inspire you! I include them here to demonstrate that the best way to reduce your risk of these cancers is to keep a lean physique. The most effective way to accomplish this is with a protein-forward diet that allows you to control hunger and maintain muscle while improving body composition through targeted physical activity.

Building Your Body Armor

When it comes to cancer, our first goal is, of course, prevention through maintaining a healthy body composition. But should a diagnosis arise, optimal body composition can offer a powerful defense. A 2016 Memorial Sloan Kettering study, for example, showed that exercise reduces the heightened risk of cardiovascular disease in women with early-stage breast cancer.[21] The more a woman exercised, the better the benefit, regardless of her age, weight, or type of cancer treatment. I've seen plenty of anecdotal evidence supporting the power of movement to reduce cancer risks as well. Over the years, I have watched many patients undergo oncology treatments and have seen how a foundation of healthy muscle mass improves outcomes. Higher muscle mass not only can support patients throughout chemotherapy and radiation, but also leads to greater survivability.

When it comes to cancer, the first thing many people think of is chemo. Rarely mentioned, however, is the cancer-induced muscle wasting that affects half of all cancer patients and plays a huge role in cancer outcomes: cancer cachexia (CC). Cachexia affects about 9 million people worldwide. This devastating syndrome is caused primarily by elevated inflammation. Eighty percent of hospitalized or advanced-stage cancer patients develop CC,[22] which ultimately becomes the immediate cause of death for at least 22 percent of cancer patients overall.[23]

Despite clear evidence to the contrary, the American Society of Clinical Oncology recently published guidelines on CC management concluding that exercise after the onset of CC is ineffective[24] and therefore not recommended. I found this not only surprising but dangerous, especially given that they were based on no trials. Even in animal CC models, resistance exercise training (RET) increases body[25] and muscle mass.[26] Moreover, RET trials in cancer patients with particularly aggressive CC forms (e.g., pancreatic cancer) already exist.[27] Notably, RET not only *did* preserve muscle mass in patients with pancreatic and lung CC,[28] but even increased body mass[29] and muscle mass[30] in patients with pancreatic CC and increased muscle mass in head and neck cancer patients undergoing radiotherapy with large (>8.5 percent) body mass loss.[31] These findings suggest that CC patients can experience clinically significant muscle mass and strength gains following supervised RET.[32] But to determine the most effective RET type and which specific exercise parameters (i.e., intensity, volume, time under tension) will simultaneously increase muscle mass and reduce inflammation, more trials are needed. It's time that mainstream medicine recognized the corrective power of healthy muscle in oncology and beyond.

Building muscle mass *before* disease strikes offers our best defense against conditions such as cachexia. But even after diagnosis, **targeted nutrition and exercise programs that promote and maintain skeletal muscle provide immediate interventions that can boost cachexia survival rates—and even help recovery.** Diet and exercise boost prevention and treatment, while survival and recovery are dependent on the underlying cause of the cachexia. Food and nutrients can be leveraged as medicine, offering powerful treatment that is both easy and accessible. Clear recognition of the pivotal role that combining key nutrients and physical activity can play in true health and survivability is the necessary first step.

Pharmacological interventions to reduce inflammation, stimulate appetite, and reduce muscle wasting already exist.[33] But far too often, the physical activity necessary to magnify the benefits of such treatments are neglected. The benefits of physical training as part of supportive cancer care are well established in the literature. Still, the medical community has yet to implement these recommendations as part of standard treatment protocols.

Patients deserve every possible defense against muscle deterioration—not just drugs. In the case of cachexia, it's important to harness the body's own ability to generate muscle through stimulus and to use patients' physical strength and capacity to push biochemical processes in a favorable direction.[34] Exercise must be doled out with the same care and precision that doctors use with any other prescription.

DEMENTIA AND ALZHEIMER'S DISEASE

Being overweight and/or obese has long been known to negatively affect memory. A large body of work shows the association between excess adipose tissue and low brain volume. Now emerging evidence has further revealed actual destruction of brain structures. By 2050, the total number of people with dementia is expected to rise to 106 million worldwide.[35] Could recognizing precursors of this debilitating condition before symptoms show help reduce that number? Recent findings suggest it might.

I saw firsthand the connection between excess fat and brain disease during my time as a fellow training in research and obesity medicine at Washington University in St. Louis. Brain scans of people in their forties revealed that a wider waistline was associated with a lower brain volume. More recent studies have confirmed these findings. One longitudinal study that measured the abdominal diameter of 6,583 individuals over time revealed that participants with the largest diameter were nearly three times more likely to develop dementia than those with the smallest diameter.[36] This means that simply being overweight exponentially increases your risk of memory loss.

Society has trained us to believe that age-related memory problems are a given. I argue, however, that memory deficits are more directly associated with low skeletal muscle than with age. If we stopped accepting waning fitness at midlife as inevitable,[37] might we see the true connection more clearly?

How Could the Size of My Waist Affect My Brain?

Just like diabetes, cardiovascular disease, and hypertension, Alzheimer's disease (AD) is, in some cases, a preventable metabolic illness. Although Alzheimer's is multifactorial and does have genetic components, my focus here is on the metabolic aspects, including the interface between weight and blood-sugar control, that contribute to brain degeneration. One way to understand AD is as type 3 diabetes of the brain.

A recent meta-analysis involving 1.3 million individuals revealed that higher BMI due to excess fat is associated with increased dementia risk when measured more than twenty years before diagnosis.[38] This means that precursors begin a full two decades before memory symptoms appear.[39] These findings have implications for a massive number of people. By 2030, 1.35 billion adults are expected to be overweight, with 573 million qualifying as obese. Interestingly, obesity has been shown to increase the risk of dementia even independently of type 2 diabetes.

The connection between girth and brain disease means much of **dementia is predictable**. People don't just wake up one day afflicted. Instead, mental decline begins with a gradual escalation over time of subtle deficits—such as challenges with word retrieval, processing information, or remembering where you left something or what you need to do next. As these changes become more obvious, they can create feelings of uneasiness and worry about increased vulnerability that can lower mood and decrease motivation. Here we see another predictable negative health outcome with impaired muscle as the root cause. Memory loss and brain destruction are among the few things in medicine that we can never undo, so prevention is the best strategy.

■

As we've now seen, again and again, healthy muscle tissue offers critical body armor against a constellation of debilitating illnesses—from cancer to cardiac disease and beyond. These disease states begin as impaired skeletal muscle that sets in motion a self-perpetuating cycle of metabolic imbalance and ill health.

We know that choices made during midlife accelerate the trajectory of aging. Losing skeletal muscle means losing the mitochondria that produce energy in your cells. It should come as no surprise that producing less energy leads to fatigue. Fatigue compounded with fewer mitochondria means you then use less energy—burning fewer of the calories that you consume. Instead, those calories get stored as fat, which leads to becoming overweight. And so the disease cycle continues.

Preserving your mitochondria by protecting skeletal muscle will help you maintain your body armor against metabolic imbalance and aging. So what are you prepared to do to grant your body the gift of health and longevity?

MINDSET RESET

SET STANDARDS TO ACHIEVE THE
HEALTH YOU DESERVE

I don't talk much about setting "goals" for wellness. To me, that framework offers too much room for failure—keeping too many people in cycles of sickness when they deserve the freedom of optimal health. Instead of goals, let's focus on setting the *standards* necessary for you to reach your future self who embodies strength, inside and out.

Social psychologist Dr. Emily Balcetis, author of *Clearer, Closer, Better: How Successful People See the World*, recommends a three-part formula for making changes: (1) dream big, (2) plan concretely, and (3) foreshadow failure.[40]

Let's break down each step.

STEP ONE: DREAM BIG

Identify WHO you want to be. WHAT qualities does that person possess? Are they fit? Are they disciplined? Are they focused? Then identify an action that embodies that future self. Dream big. Define what success would look like for you. Envision the ACTION or HABIT that will get you there.

STEP TWO: MAKE CONCRETE PLANS

Implement a protocol like the ones in this book. Break down plan execution into small steps:

1. Schedule the grocery shopping.
2. Plan when you'll cook.
3. Prepack your meals for the day.

Identify all the logistical tasks that you need to do TODAY to instill the habits that narrow the gap between your present and future selves. Take these same steps again tomorrow, the next day, and each day thereafter. Big progress comes from moving forward in small increments—not only in your health but in making over your mental framework.

STEP THREE: FORESHADOW FAILURE

What energy sinks will draw your focus away from execution? Where are the daily pitfalls of focus and energy that will prevent you from achieving the standards you've set? This requires awareness of your personal weaknesses. Some examples:

- Did you skip your run because you couldn't tolerate losing forty minutes of sleep? Those minutes could have helped to ramp up your energy and clear your head for a fresh start to the day.
- Did you miss your evening workout because your job left you dead tired and desperate to "zone out" in front of a screen? Bringing your binge-watch to the elliptical might have been the movement push you needed to follow through with your training program.
- Did you forgo the gym in favor of the drinks you felt you deserved as a Friday afternoon wind-down? Imagine how much better Saturday morning would have felt if you'd

woken up not queasy from overindulging but pleasantly sore from training.

These what-if scenarios all paint scenes of predictable traps of human nature along with counterforce alternatives. Succumbing to impulses that impede action will kill any health goal. So choose awareness instead. Consider the obstacles you'll face, and come to expect them. Instead of veering, predictably, off course, visualize a new strategy BEFORE you end up in a compromising position.

Raising yourself up to high standards takes hard work and planning. Keep reminding yourself of the costs of continuing your negative habits while cultivating the positivity that will propel you to execute. Our ultimate goal is for the health-promoting action to become so well practiced and ingrained that it becomes your default response—creating a life that supports your own vision for yourself.

Speaking of that vision . . . did you know that building muscle can help you reach age-specific goals?

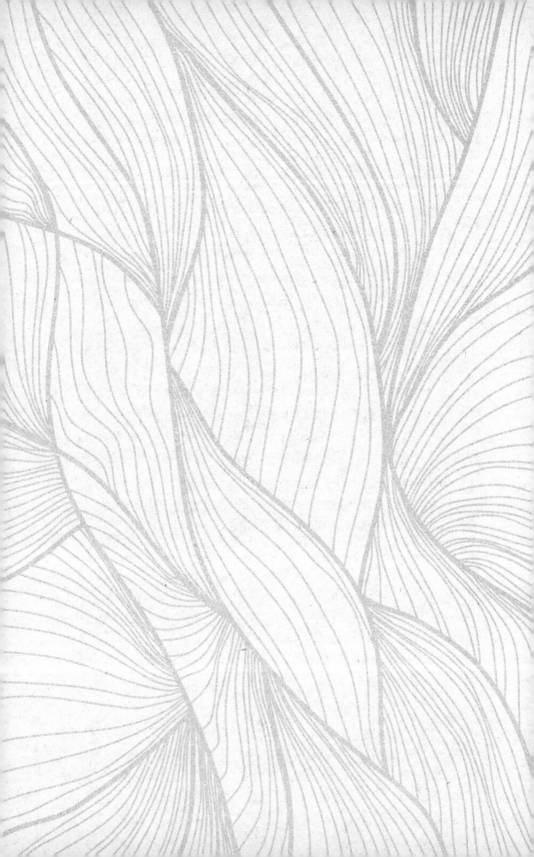

3.

~~~~~

Bulletproof Your Changing Body
for Strength at Every Age

We age every day. Every single one of us. None of us is immune to that reality. But the choices we make based on the knowledge we have will greatly determine the quality and trajectory of our lives, now and in the future. The first step is establishing a healthy framework for viewing getting older. As a trained geriatrician, I will tell you from experience that what matters is the QUALITY of life you can maintain over the years. Even if you don't develop a major illness, when it comes to the activities of daily living, nothing determines your life quality more than muscle health. Mobility is essential to preserving your own autonomy and ability to do what you enjoy. Metabolic health drives the strength and vigor of your body's functions system-wide.

As we get older, so much gets better and stronger—our mental resilience, our problem-solving skills, the depths of our relationships—but at the same time, our bodies are steadily losing power inside and out. By planning for the natural, predictable changes that occur with time, we can commit to the nutritional and training strategies that will counter all sorts of declines. Have doubts? Consider lifelong athletes who, at age seventy, have more and healthier muscle tissue than lots of people half their age.

Recognizing the innate physiological processes that impact our well-being allows us to influence the factors we can, taking charge of our own longevity in powerful ways. The first step forward is learning to decipher your body's changes to elevate your understanding about *why* to implement the strategies I recommend. We often think of disease states as binary—you either have an illness or you don't. Instead, a more typical evolution is like a low, smoldering flame that will grow into a full-blown forest fire if left unchecked. The longer you let the fire build, the harder it becomes to ever recover from the damage. Aging does not mean we all have to become less conditioned. But we do have to work smarter and with more intention and focus on staying Forever Strong.

START YOUNG

Remember, the game of life is survival of the strongest. Both nutritional and physical literacy—knowing what to eat and how to move—are imperative, and it's never too early to start. Society's obsession with adult obesity spills over into our concerns about children. But the focus on fat over muscle continues to lead us astray. Building and maintaining healthy muscle tissue is critical for young people, too, and targeting muscle development early on lays the foundation for longevity.

According to the CDC, childhood obesity rates have tripled over the past three decades, affecting 20 percent of children ages two to nineteen, or about 14.7 million. Between 2001 and 2017, the number of people younger than twenty living with type 2 diabetes grew by 95 percent, according to CDC data.[1] The American Academy of Pediatrics says that a poor diet increases a child's risk of diabetes—which is associated with hypertension, sleep apnea, fatty liver disease, and depression—explaining that it's one of the most common pediatric chronic diseases.[2] Meanwhile, data from the 2021 National Survey of Children's Health showed that in a given week, 32 percent of children did not eat a daily fruit, 49 percent did not eat a daily vegetable, and 57 percent drank a sugar-sweetened beverage at least once. Given all we know about how a proper diet supports optimal growth and health, **how could we let the nutrition bar drop so low?**

Just like in banking, early investment in muscle health reaps rewards that compound over time. Resistance exercise and nutrient-rich foods prepare a young person to reach their full physical and mental potential—not to mention boosting their body awareness and helping them feel self-confident and powerful. Exercise is, of course, crucial for cardiovascular health in young people. Equally important, although often overlooked in children and adolescents, are the benefits of muscular fitness, characterized by strength, power, and local muscular endurance.[3] Each of us is born with a certain number of muscle fibers,[4] but whether we actualize our muscle's potential by growing those fibers and creating new ones from satellite (stem) cells depends on our dedication to physical fitness throughout our lifetime. Because your body has muscle memory, putting down a deposit on strength is valuable, positively influencing the key regulatory genes involved in muscle adaptations to resistance exercise.[5]

Resistance training is safe and effective for children and adolescents, according to the American Academy of Pediatrics, leading to improvements in health, fitness, injury reduction, and rehabilitation, as well as physical literacy.[6] Not limited to lifting weights, resistance exercise can incorporate a wide array of body-weight movements, including fun exercises such as frog jumps, bear crawls, crab walks, and kangaroo or one-leg hops. Contrary to the outdated myth that kids can't lift weights, resistance training is for everybody at any age.

Well-supervised, fun-focused training that emphasizes proper technique is a safe way to spark an ongoing interest in exercise. Strength training in kids increases capacity for motor-neuron recruitment, offering lifelong benefits. The key is to build from a solid form foundation, making sure a child can successfully perform the baseline movements needed before adding load. More serious weightlifting, beyond five- to ten-pound dumbbells, can begin during puberty.

Because young people exist in a hormone-driven growth phase, muscle tissue is much more responsive at an early age. Strength training performed safely at developmentally appropriate levels lays groundwork that lasts a lifetime. While this book is not specifically geared toward kids, it's critical to consider how the Lyon Protocol lays out sound principles for eating and exercise that can benefit the whole family. The more physically active a child is, the more protein may be beneficial for their growth.[7]

Of all factors that we can manipulate, diet in infancy and early childhood is among the most influential. Providing our kids with nutritious, whole foods balanced in macronutrients can set them up for healthy development, a lean body composition, and habits that can nurture them through adolescence and into adulthood.[8] Low-protein diets during these critical years can impede growth and cause fatigue during sports and active play. A protein-forward diet in youth, on the other hand, provides the fuel our kids need to learn, grow, thrive, and challenge themselves—as well as helping to prevent metabolic disasters later in life. We know the effects of healthy muscle are cumulative. That's why we need to establish early strength training as standard protocol for all our children.

Did you know that while your child is learning how to climb the monkey bars or pull themselves up a climbing wall, they're changing the nature and capacity of their muscle cells? We often use the phrase "muscle memory" figuratively, but recent findings reveal how **muscle really does attain and retain memory on a cellular level**, through exercise-induced increases in myonuclei.[9]

Research showing that previously trained muscle has a greater number of myonuclei suggests that starting resistance training early allows muscle tissue to obtain "cellular memory" through this increase. Muscle fibers that have a higher number of myonuclei grow faster, especially when exposed to resistance exercise in the future.[10]

START NOW!

Contrary to what many assume, the aging we are talking about—the **inevitable physiological changes to muscle and overall body composition—begins in our thirties.** Starting to build muscle while you're young allows you to build your biological reserve, the effects of which will stay with you for a lifetime. After all, older people's ability to maintain strength and muscle mass is determined not only by the *rate of loss* but also by the *starting point* from which that loss begins, that is, the peak muscle mass reached earlier in life.[11] Choices made early on direct the system, ultimately determining energy, vitality, and staying power.

That said, **it is never too late to start.** Positive changes may not come as quickly, but I promise you will see improvements. The steps you take right now—TODAY!—can rewrite your future.

Bottom line: the healthier your muscle mass, the greater your chances of living and thriving.

TWENTIES AND THIRTIES

When you're in your twenties and thirties, it might seem like you can get away with fad diets and cycling through juice cleanses—that you can chase every latest nutrition trend that convinces you to stockpile supplements, load up on "super" foods, decide to go vegan, or push the boundaries of going all plant-based at the expense of protein.[12] But sometimes too much information is not a good thing. My approach is to home in on what the science recommends over the long haul rather than let you get caught up in the latest craze.

Spoiler alert: quick fixes never work. Instead, following my step-by-step Lyon Protocol will establish a solid foundation upon which to build a future of strength, good health, and longevity. The health benefits of a physically active lifestyle during adolescence and early adulthood aren't just physical. There is also growing evidence that exercise has a positive impact on cognitive development, socializing, stress reduction, and an overall sense of mental well-being.

During early adulthood, your hormones reach their peak, with testosterone, growth hormone, and insulin-like growth factor 1 (IGF-1) primed for growth. Maybe, on a superficial level, you can get away with less discipline while these hormones are running high; your body will do its best with whatever nutrition you give it. But relying on a youth-dependent get-out-of-jail-free card can set you up for long-term bad habits. Instead, with diligence and focused attention, you can establish patterns of behavior that will serve you both now and in the long run.

Here's a sobering bit of information that should help get you on track toward good health, despite the seemingly forgiving nature of your twenty- or thirtysomething-year-old self. **You will likely reach your peak bone mass between age twenty-five and thirty.** Bone health is determined in large part by muscle strength and the communication between these organ systems. There is a clear positive correlation between lean body mass and bone density.[13] You know how peaks work, right? Once you reach the top, it's downhill from there. Why not set yourself up for the best possible descent?

CINDY'S STORY

One of my patients, a biologist named Cindy, had always been into fitness yet struggled to gain muscle. She was thin, with low muscle mass, and had what some would describe as a skinny-fat physique. When she transitioned from fieldwork to a desk job, she wound up sitting all day, struggling with fatigue. She kept her calories in check but wound up eating mostly highly processed, fake Frankenfoods that provided low nutrient density. Her health was further compromised by a slew of environmental exposures from the reduced quality of water and both indoor and outdoor air. In Cindy's case, the regular exposures of daily American life were compounded by toxic mold in her home.

Cindy might have been fed, but she was undernourished, due to a diet lacking in fiber and whole foods. Low iron and zinc levels had left her hair and nails brittle and breaking. Her long sessions of steady-state cardio at the gym took up lots of time but had little impact. Cindy had fallen into an all-too-common trap. Like so many other women afraid of "bulking up," she had never given strength training a second thought.

To turn her life around, I created a structure to her diet, establishing clear, consistent mealtimes. I increased her protein, shifted her focus away from eating solely low-calorie packaged food, and centered her diet on whole nutrient-dense foods that nourished her body. **Her transformation reminded me of a wilted flower suddenly given water.** She gained muscle and started hitting new personal-best records for strength. Her energy bounced from a level two to a ten. No longer reliant on constant caffeine infusion, she was able to reduce her morning coffee intake from four cups to just one. Her blood markers improved, including her iron stores. Her hair, skin, and nails glowed. She also was able to manage food cravings by concentrating attention on her desire for overall wellness. No longer crashing at 3 p.m., she could hardly believe the energy that was possible with her new normal.

Once I gave her clear guidance, Cindy became a star patient—a queen of execution. She thrived on a clear food strategy of carefully balanced macros that corrected her diet's nutrient density. I also altered her workout strategy and gave her tools to get her sleep back on track. The change was profound. Her tank now filled with the macro- and micronutrients she needed, Cindy's energy levels exploded. Her mood no longer tanked around her period, nor was she filled with fear whenever she ate carbs, like so many young women I see today. She nourished rather than restricting her body. She put on muscle without getting bulky and shed body fat despite being "skinny," so much so that she entered her first bikini show, now having the confidence to step onstage in a swimsuit. Weight loss wasn't her goal. Just complete transformation—and it happened.

FERTILITY

Infertility, along with both obesity and overweight, is on the rise not only in Western countries but worldwide. Often thought of as solely a matter of hormones, fertility is, in truth, tightly linked to diet and lifestyle in both men and women. In turn, body leanness plays a unique, important role in the optimization, maximization, and objective markers of health that drive fertility.

Female Infertility

Generally defined as *failure to conceive after twelve or more months of attempts of natural fertilization*, infertility affects between 50 million and 80 million women, according to World Health Organization (WHO) estimates.[14] The most common cause of female infertility in women of childbearing age is failing to ovulate, which occurs in 40 percent of women with fertility issues.[15] Obesity is known to disrupt female fertility, and even being slightly overweight can be associated with decreased pregnancy rates.[16]

One challenge that confronts as many as 5 million women in the US—approximately 6 to 12 percent of women of reproductive age—is polycystic ovary syndrome (PCOS), which is linked to insulin resistance, muscle tissue differences, and often sarcopenic obesity later in life.[17] This condition directly affects muscle tissue, causing reduced insulin-mediated glucose uptake and sometimes defects in insulin signaling. PCOS is often thought of as related to obesity, but affected individuals have significant peripheral insulin resistance, separate from BMI. Even lean women with PCOS have higher levels of intramuscular fat, which may be the cause of their reduced insulin sensitivity. Independent of obesity, people with PCOS have decreased ability to dispose of glucose. Skeletal muscle is one focal point of treatment. This emphasizes the key role of high-intensity exercise in reversing problems of insulin resistance.[18] Improving fertility depends not only on mitigating the effects of carrying excess fat but also on addressing insulin issues at a molecular level. Exercise and nutrition can be used to amplify cell signaling that helps with both. It's now more than clear that muscle needs to be recognized as a focal point for understanding one of the most common causes of infertility in women.[19]

Pregnancy

Skeletal muscle is a hero for a healthy pregnancy. This remarkable organ system can adapt to the normal changes that occur when a woman carries a child, allowing the fetus access to essential nutrients while buffering the impact of those changes on the mother. A healthy pregnancy changes metabolism, hormones, and blood circulation. It also creates a form of insulin resistance, by design. Research shows that insulin-mediated whole-body glucose disposal decreases by 50 percent in pregnancy.[20]

We've already discussed the dangers of insulin resistance. Why would this be an expected part of the gestational process? For a very good reason. Pregnancy increases the mother's blood glucose and free fatty acids to make these nutrients available to the fetus. This means you will have higher blood glucose just from being pregnant. Women with a healthy, normal glucose tolerance can manage the shift by increasing insulin production. But when the mother's body can't make and use all the insulin it needs, the glucose remains in the bloodstream, which leads to high blood sugar and ultimately gestational diabetes. Nearly 10 percent of pregnancies in the US are affected by gestational diabetes each year.[21] While treatable, this condition raises high-blood-pressure risk in the mother and can hurt the baby as well. Gestational diabetes increases the risk of a baby being born large (nine pounds or more) and complicating delivery; a premature birth, which can cause breathing and other problems; having low blood sugar at birth; and developing type 2 diabetes later in life.

The best defense—for you and your baby—is to go into pregnancy as fit as you can be. If you begin your pregnancy journey sedentary or with already insulin-resistant skeletal muscle, you are starting from a disadvantaged health state.[22] With rising rates of obesity, more women are going into pregnancy overweight, unhealthy, and at increased risk because they're already metabolically compromised.[23]

The role of healthy skeletal muscle in protecting both mother and child has been grossly overlooked. Insulin resistance in pregnancy is normal, but gestational diabetes is not.[24] Healthy skeletal muscle can help protect mothers from developing gestational diabetes, and studies make clear the importance of both resistance and aerobic exercise in improving blood-glucose levels.[25] The key is incorporating more muscle activity into any perinatal training program.

Male Infertility

Fat decreases testosterone by converting it to estrogen in excess adipose tissue and unhealthy, marbled muscle. It also leads to the blood-sugar problems we've already highlighted, which increases cortisol levels that decrease fertility in men.

On the brighter side, **muscle contraction may positively affect reproduction**. By improving hormone production and response, improving body composition, and regulating inflammatory responses in the body, muscle health improves fertility. Mounting evidence suggests that different types of training interventions can successfully improve several aspects of male reproductive function among both fertile and infertile men.[26] In fact, exercise has been shown to improve the quantity and quality of viable sperm as well as increasing semen volume.[27] If fat is fouling up fertility, growing more healthy muscle, which will improve your metabolism, can help.

LATE THIRTIES TO EARLY FORTIES

D r. Lyon, I don't know what happened. I eat and exercise like I always have, but now I keep gaining weight." I hear this almost daily from my patients in this age group. This is absolutely predictable, common, and to be expected. Thirty- to fortysomething-year-olds have reached the ultimate metabolic turning point, and signs will begin to appear on your body and potentially in your bloodwork. One thing is for certain: seeing changes on the outside increases the likelihood that

you're carrying unhealthy skeletal muscle on the inside. If you continue to eat and train like the typical twentysomething-year-old, you
will start to put on fat and further push the envelope of muscle-health
decline. Fortunately, by following evidence-based principles, you can
correct the behaviors that exacerbate age-driven metabolic changes. **If
you missed the window when you were younger, this is your golden
moment. Take this decade to focus on building the body protection
you need.**

You don't need to wait for the future to experience the benefits
of working on your health today. Sure, body composition correction
will give you the lift of seeing a rebalance in your bloodwork. But you
will also *feel better* every day. **Metabolic health allows for better sleep
and increased energy.** At a moment when your hormones are peak-
ing, **healthy muscle will make you mentally stronger, turbocharging
your ability to shine at work,** at a time when career building is often
of paramount concern. Muscle-centric living can even **boost your love
life, helping you become more flexible and feel better naked.** Plus,
exercise has been shown to increase libido.

All these effects can ripple out to those around you. Did you know
research suggests that obesity can "spread" within social networks?
(A 2007 study showed that if one friend became obese during a given
time interval, the other friend's chances of following suit increased by
171 percent.)[28] The same can be said for the "spread" of human health.
How you execute raises the wellness bar for those around you.

Can you guess the key element for arming yourself against age-
related decline? Of course, it's protein (and resistance training)! As you
transitioned from high school to college or work, old habits probably
trailed behind you, barking at your heels. Once the period of physical
growth ends, we need to make smart changes to optimize body
composition and maintain good health. This is the crucial moment

for understanding and maximizing the vital capacity of muscle as a nutrient-sensing organ—one of the most potent pathways toward muscle growth and health.

MID- TO LATE FORTIES

Aging is inevitable. We all do it, all day, every day. Explaining muscle as a fountain of youth is not to deny or disparage the realities of getting older. Instead, I want to help us confront directly the inevitable, predictable transformations that happen over time, so we can work them to our best advantage.

Sick of gaining and losing the same ten pounds? Desperate for a solid night of uninterrupted sleep? Wish you could make it to 3 p.m. without dragging yourself through the remainder of your day? Struggling with brain fog, word retrieval, or feeling demoralized? I'm here to tell you, relief is in sight! Right here, right now, is your opportunity to seize control of your health rather than allowing the aging process to take away your freedom.

We know that muscle's ability to sense nutrients diminishes with age. When muscle becomes less responsive to protein—particularly low doses of amino acids—the tissue changes. When these changes occur, the metabolic abilities of the muscle tissue significantly decline, increasing our risks for disease, fatigue, and obesity. Once tissue destruction begins (which can happen at any age but is generally detectable in one's forties), combating the inevitable weight-loss and health struggles becomes more of a challenge.

Obesity impairs muscle by creating a toxic metabolic environment in the muscle. Toxic fat by-products overpack our skeletal-muscle suitcase, leaving us weak, less flexible, and unable to efficiently process the food calories that we eat. The deposit of lipids into skeletal muscle impairs muscle's ability to contract, while interfering with the synthesis of amino acids into new healthy muscle tissue. Fat accumulation does not just build up in fat cells but spreads into muscle. This makes it more difficult to recover from exercise or injury as well as blunting the ability to lay down more muscle.

Because compromised muscle is less responsive to protein, adults older than forty require a nutrition plan that prioritizes turning on muscle-protein synthesis (MPS)—*the processing of amino acids into skeletal muscle.* Don't worry. I'll explain this whole process in much greater depth in chapter 5. Until then, rest assured that the inescapable metabolic realities of getting older are built into my plan to help you over the long haul.

The Lyon Protocol also accounts for changes in muscle insulin resistance. While reduced regenerative capacity is just a reality, that doesn't mean there aren't other changes within your direct control that will impact your vitality. Consider this the make-or-break decade. The highlight reel for this period shows shot after shot of body fat because that what's visible on the surface. Hidden from view, however, is a more subtle effect: the slow, quiet destruction of muscle.

Without proper diet and resistance training, deterioration of skeletal muscle mass (sarcopenia) and declines in strength and power (dynapenia) that begin in your thirties usually wind up quite noticeable by age fifty. These reductions occur at a rate of around 0.8 to 1 percent and around 2 to 3 percent per year, respectively. This trajectory leads to muscle loss combined with body-fat gain that results in sarcopenia AND obesity, known as sarcopenic obesity. Both sarcopenia and obesity reflect poor metabolic health. Sarcopenic obesity, therefore, may result in an even greater risk of metabolic disorders and fatal cardiovascular disease.[29]

That's why exercising isn't just a vanity thing. If you stop moving, your muscle starts shrinking. One study showed around a 3 percent decrease in leg-muscle tissue after just seven days of bed rest in older adults.[30] (Yikes!) While you might dismiss bed rest as something that only affects the ill or aging, anyone **who becomes sick, inactive, *or simply stops training* is at risk of significant muscle tissue decline.** Bed rest is not a benign treatment without side effects. In fact, it causes potentially more harm than good. Recommended to nearly all patients entering the hospital, despite the results of a 1999 systematic review that found no benefits for any of the seventeen conditions studied,[31] bed rest is a largely outdated practice. Here we see another consequence of the full metabolic power of muscle going largely unrecognized in mainstream medicine. Immobilizing people in bed when most of us are already starting off with insufficient lean muscle mass is a potentially harmful "treatment" in need of more careful examination.

Unless you've been a lifelong athlete who's consistently prioritized protein and muscle building, chances are you could use more healthy muscle mass. Recent estimates indicate that 8 percent to 36 percent of individuals younger than sixty and from 10 percent to 27 percent of those sixty or older are considered sarcopenic. Severe sarcopenia among those in the sixty-plus category ranged from 2 percent to 9 percent.[32] By the fifth decade of life, metabolism improvement becomes significantly more difficult, but the window of wellness opportunity never closes completely. At this age, if you eat the proper quantity, quality, and distribution of protein and train aggressively (see chapters 5 and 9) to heal and build your muscle, you can reverse metabolic dysfunction and, depending on your current metrics, build back pounds of muscle within months. So it's time to get to work!

It's never too late to get Forever Strong.

"Remember, age is the great equalizer. Your habits determine how you navigate maturity."

FIFTIES

Getting older brings us maturity, perspective, and sometimes even wisdom! Plus, research conducted over a twenty-year span showed that many of us feel less stress as we age.[33] Still, Father Time also challenges us with the loss of skeletal-muscle mass. After about age fifty, muscle mass decreases at an annual rate of 1 to 2 percent.[34] Often the lost muscle is replaced by body fat, reducing muscle strength and mobility while also disrupting metabolism.

The decline in muscle strength is even higher. A perfect storm of reduced activity, subpar nutrition, hormone decreases, injury, and inflammation often plays a role. But unlike with the weather, we can change the forces that create these declines. We can blunt the loss of both muscle mass and strength by making smart choices about dietary protein and resistance exercise. As I've mentioned, older adults need more dietary protein to support good health, promote recovery from illness, and maintain functionality.

BENEFITS OF A HIGHER PROTEIN INTAKE FOR OLDER ADULTS

→ Higher bone density

→ Slower rate of bone loss

→ Slower rate of muscle loss

→ Increased resilience

Pairing optimal protein intake with resistance training maintains muscle health and works to help address dysfunctional eating behaviors, fatty liver disease, obesity, hypertension, hyperglycemia, and high cholesterol, along with preventing many other diseases. By teaching people about the power of protein, I'm able to frame the nutritional solutions that finally make the difference. Time and again, I've helped my patients succeed at making these life-altering changes.

Health-care professionals can argue all they want about eating less protein and more vegetables while people are young or in midlife, but the argument ends there. No respected geriatrician will say that eating a low-protein diet or sacrificing muscle mass is safe for the mature adult population. Sarcopenia's slow decrease in skeletal-muscle mass that contributes to the risk of chronic diseases is a direct predictor of disability. Our goal must be to gain and maintain as much muscle mass as possible to prepare for this inevitable decline. Fortunately, even aging muscle remains plastic, meaning improvement is always possible.

Menopause

Just about every woman in or approaching menopause can attest to the body-fat distribution changes that occur during this period. As estrogen and progesterone production decline with menopause, their relative imbalance compared to cortisol further exacerbates insulin resistance. These hormone shifts, combined with a decrease in energy expenditure, can cause weight gain. But *can* does not mean *will*. **Excess fat and decreased muscle health are not inevitable!**

As your progesterone and estrogen start to decrease, you can counter the effects of these hormone declines with the powerful stimuli offered by dietary intervention and focused cardio and resistance training. The tools for mitigating menopausal changes are in your hands, under your direct, voluntary control. How cool is that?

The most common struggle women have during this transition is an almost immediate large gain in fat and decrease in muscle mass. This affects self-confidence, emotional well-being, and overall quality of life. Countless times, I've heard women give up, saying, "I am just old now. This is how my body will look from now on, and there is no point in trying." The reality couldn't be farther from the truth.

Once you understand the changes that happen as hormonal shifts occur, you can create a plan that allows to you win in any hormonal situation. Perimenopause is the time to really dial in your mental framework, hone your high-intensity interval training (HIIT) (see more on page 233), and optimize protein intake, while moderating carbohydrate consumption—particularly post-workout and around bedtime. Taking these steps will set you up with a strong, healthy metabolic baseline of lean-muscle mass that will help you weather the coming changes.

Menopause brings about a rapid decline in estrogen, which leads to more testosterone dominance. Postmenopausal ovaries become androgen-secreting organs, producing roughly 25 percent of the body's testosterone. It's not that more overall testosterone gets produced at this time but rather that decreased estrogen provides less counterforce against the androgen's effects. While estrogen distributes weight to women's hips and butt, testosterone encourages fat around the midsection. This transition expresses itself with a sudden decrease in muscle mass and bone density, as well as increased risk of truncal obesity.

Research suggests that estrogen in women impacts both function and hypertrophy (building increased mass) of skeletal muscle.[35] As estrogen levels drop, the skeletal-muscle organ system that had previously been supported by youthful estrogen levels begins to decline. Because estrogen offers critical support for tendons and ligaments, menopausal decline increases the risk of injury and joint pain. This same effect can be observed in women taking birth control pills that suppress natural hormone production.

The vulnerability of this period is exacerbated by erratic food intake. I see many women struggle from the effects of the cantaloupe lunch and a small chicken-breast salad and mocha latté for dinner, combined with their standard training of walking, Zumba, or Pilates. This is not the strong medicine we need to fortify menopausal women for their future.

Instead, a muscle-centric lifestyle involving a higher-protein diet designed around balanced macros and a strict calorie budget combined with the rigorous resistance training that will turn that protein into muscle can keep you strong, healthy, and energized throughout menopause.

KIM'S STORY

At sixty-three, Kim was incredibly active. She had been following a ketogenic diet for several years and lifted weights regularly. After hitting menopause a decade earlier, Kim had begun hormone-replacement therapy. She typically fasted until midday. Then she kept to a strict low-carb and ketogenic diet. Still, she started to gain belly fat, noticed hair loss, and struggled to put on muscle, despite lifting weights three times a week. She came to me for help fine-tuning her plan. "I have listened to all your interviews," she said, presenting me with the macros breakdown she'd put together by following the Lyon Protocol. "Walk me through all the details to make sure I am doing everything correctly so I can age amazingly." Although she had come to me with excellent muscle health overall, her balance of exercise and dietary protein needed tweaking.

First we tackled her diet. Her keto-based nutrition was too high in fat and too low in protein to keep up with the metabolic changes of aging. This left her unable to trigger the muscle-growth response—until I restructured her eating program. I stopped her fasting and switched her from a ketogenic to a higher-protein diet. We increased her protein to 80 grams a day (approximately 1.6 grams per kilogram) to offset her muscle loss. We added in creatine and branched-chain amino acids (BCAAs), as well as a specifically timed whey-protein shake. The goal of supplementation was to keep her calories low while supporting brain and muscle health with creatine and fueling muscle synthesis with BCAAs. Plus, because she was no longer training as hard as she had in her forties, we added an essential amino acid drink to further bump up her protein intake without any extra calories she would have needed to burn off in the gym. Following her program to a T, she put on three pounds of muscle within the first month.

Increasing the volume and focus of her training helped too. We cut back her cardio and had her use that time on exercises that pushed her to muscle failure and fatigue. Kim learned to push herself through two days of full-body strength training, plus a day of upper body and another of lower body. She also learned how satisfying it felt to go hard. We were able to halt the pattern of muscle loss, helping her gain half a pound of muscle every two months or so. By halting her fasting, reducing her fat, adding appropriate supplements, targeting her protein, and shifting up her training, she improved phenomenally.

ANDROPAUSE

Women aren't the only ones who experience age-related hormonal changes. Testosterone decrease—a natural, expected part of men's aging process—causes a reduction in muscle and an increase in fat that can lead to an imbalance in body composition and a rise in the diseases that follow declining muscle health.

Testosterone improves muscle-protein synthesis, which helps prevent muscle tissue breakdown and protects against cardiovascular disease. These functions become increasingly important with age or if we face health challenges. As part of growing muscle mass and strength, testosterone raises the number of satellite cells available to promote normal growth, repair, and regeneration. Without stimulation from resistance training, these cells can enter a "pause" or dormant state, and the longer they stay inactive, the harder they are to reactivate. Stimulating these cells through exercise can protect against dormancy and mitigate muscle decline.[36]

In other words, a man who prioritizes resistance training as he gets older can prevent the "pause" of satellite cells and in turn possess muscle that is more highly equipped to repair itself and to grow in size and strength. Conversely, the muscle in a man who remains sedentary through the aging process will not have these regenerative and growth capacities. As a result, he will end up with weaker, more insulin-resistant muscles.

This creates a starting point that can lead to a cascade of additional problems. Unlike menopause, which has a clear point of cessation, andropause (low testosterone) proceeds over decades. Outside of lab results, how can you know if you are suffering from low testosterone? Look out for low libido, difficulty putting on muscle, or an increase in belly fat. All of these can be signs of andropause. Remember, while getting older is inevitable, the health declines caused by diminished muscle mass are NOT! **A muscle-centric lifestyle incorporating nutritional and movement changes can rewrite your life story.**

SIXTY AND OLDER

Beyond sixty, you will reap the rewards of the habits you've culti-vated toward strength and committed physical effort. Your muscles have cellular memory, so a nervous system that has been well trained for movement is primed to protect you. If your wellness habits have, so far, been less than stellar, the striking loss of muscle mass and other shifts in body composition might just be the wake-up call you need to execute real change—starting today! Because this is a time when chronic disuse and injuries can crop up and limit mobility, taking in-formed steps toward fortifying yourself, inside and out, is an essential part of building a foundation of healthy practices that will serve you throughout the rest of your life.

For people older than sixty, quality of life becomes the primary consideration for any diet and exercise plan. I'll say it again: **the best way to safeguard your independence is to protect your skeletal-muscle mass.** According to the CDC, 3 million older people are treated in emergency departments annually for falls. Each year, one in three adults older than sixty-five falls. One-quarter of those who suffer a hip fracture die in the following year, and the most common cause of accidental death in people older than sixty-five is fall-related injury.[37] You don't have to be included in these statistics!

Research shows that a well-designed resistance-training program of two to four days a week successfully increases maximal strength, muscle mass, muscle power, and functional capacity among individu-als older than sixty-five. Other studies highlight the cognitive benefits of cardio and resistance training for people in this age group, citing the brain-boosting, body-awareness benefits of the feel-good hormones that the combination of these types of exercise releases.[38] While im-provements won't happen as quickly as starting when you're younger, a well-designed program can bring you these benefits even if you begin exercising later in life.

Because not many people fall off cliffs and die, fall-death counts seem minor when it comes to an official cause of death. In actuality, however, muscle health and mobility issues underlie at least nine of the top ten "causes" of death. To put this in perspective, obesity is also not listed as a major cause of death according to the CDC. Yet it is the underlying condition leading to heart disease, cancer, diabetes, respiratory stress, Alzheimer's, and more. Obesity and muscle health and mobility are all leading factors in mortality, but the CDC has no way to quantify the relationship. They only report what a doctor puts on a death certificate.

In the aftermath of a fall, maintaining activities of daily living (ADL) can become a major health problem that affects everything from cognitive and emotional well-being to metabolic health. More than 300,000 adults in the US above age sixty-five get hospitalized annually for hip fractures. This sets the stage for a catabolic crisis to occur in the years that follow. "Heart disease" deaths in the US total about 380,000 per year. Another 320,000 die because their heart stops (reason unknown). If we consider falls through this lens of catabolic crisis, they become a leading cause of injury and death for people aged sixty-five and up, and the second-leading cause of unintentional death worldwide.[39] Skeletal muscle is your body armor in the battle of life!

I'll never sugarcoat the actual scientific processes that make it harder to repair damaged muscle. But I will tell you, in no uncertain terms, that **IT IS NEVER TOO LATE TO IMPROVE YOUR MUSCLE HEALTH!**

Even if illness, injury, or just plain old life has left you less active than you should be, you can get stronger and fitter and enjoy a burst of newfound energy. Even if you're nursing an injury, there are countless work-arounds to increase your activity level in a safe, controlled way. It helps to take any emotional negotiation out of the equation. Simply tell yourself today is the day you'll begin training (for the first time or again). Sure, you might not start out with the same strength and agility as you wish you had, or had once before, but do not let a defeatist attitude stand in your way. Instead, choose something doable that will make you feel good. The goal is to avoid beating yourself up about any decline in favor of inspiring yourself to keep going.

MINDSET RESET

OVERCOMING PRESENT BIAS

We track our time, our money, our calories, but rarely do we take time to track and organize our complex minds. Your inherent nature has been affecting your health all along. I'm here to give you a working model for creating the mental organization and control to build the body you deserve. With this scaffolding in place, we can now anticipate the obstacles you're likely to encounter on the proverbial battlefield. One of the hardest to conquer is present bias.

The human tendency toward **present bias prioritizes our current wants and desires over our long-term personal goals.** Essentially, we make choices that favor our present selves over our future selves. Present bias embodies the struggle of procrastination—putting off until tomorrow the actions that need to be taken today. I see examples of present bias all too often in clinic. Despite desperately wanting to lose fat and gain lean, healthy muscle, some of my patients struggle to stick with the consistent diet they know will serve them best in the future. Rather than focusing on how their actions will affect their long-term health goals, they wind up giving in to their immediate desires for the cookies, the bottle of wine, or the bag of chips.

Present bias is a hardwired tendency that leads humans to give in to short-term desires at the expense of long-term outcomes. This phenomenon involves two different players, the current self and the future self, and the divide between them can be huge. Both the current self and the future self are parts of you. The one you nurture more will dominate the other.

Here's an example. My patient Maria, mother of three, felt like her body never recovered after kids. For three years, she'd been struggling to lose twenty pounds. "I really want to lose weight, and I am so structured during the day. Then, at night when my girls are having cookies, I eat them, too," she said. "I tell myself I'll do better tomorrow."

That tomorrow did not come for Maria for at least three years. This is a prime example of letting your present self win out over your future self. Let's break down how this happens. Making self-defeating choices like this involves opting for a smaller reward of enjoying treats in the immediate term over the bigger reward of being in great shape in the future. By succumbing to cookies, Maria is trying to alleviate the discomfort and pressure of doing what she doesn't want to do.

Psychologically speaking, there could be many reasons. Maybe her self-worth temperature is low. (See page 219 to gauge your own self-worth level.) Maybe she doesn't feel she deserves to lose weight. Maybe she has a habit of turning to food for emotional comfort. Whether conscious or unconscious, the present-self script she's running is undermining her future dreams and sabotaging her life. On a very primal level, this is not her fault. We all have a present self that we must do battle with to get what we really want in life.

Maria and I had a pretty tough heart-to-heart about how her present self was sabotaging her future self, and finally it clicked. First, I introduced her to her future self—that part of Maria who is disciplined and fit and who understands that to keep this future self, she must collapse the distance between now and later. She must allow her future self to be stronger than her present self. This is where the real training comes in—not with weights but in the mind.

Together we got very clear about who she wanted to be and outlined the step-by-step actions that would take her there. Then we put in consequences as a way of establishing guardrails. What worked for Maria was this: every time she let her present self eat the cookies, she would take a stack of twenty singles and throw them out the window of her car. That stung. She hated the waste, so this was a perfect consequence for stepping out of integrity with her future self. Guess how many times she had to follow through with that consequence? Once. It took one time to change the habit forever. Through establishment of appropriate guardrails combined with fostering a tight connection with her future self, we were able to collapse the two selves so Maria could finally reach her goals.

FUTURE PROJECTION

People often suggest that you visualize what you want and how it will feel when you get it. Here's what I've found works better: do a future projection of what it will *cost* you if you hang on to your current bad habits. This is incredibly effective. It highlights what you will have to give up if you continue to make negative choices.

Sit in a quiet place and imagine . . .

If you continue these negative practices going forward, what will it cost you in two years? How about four? How about twenty?

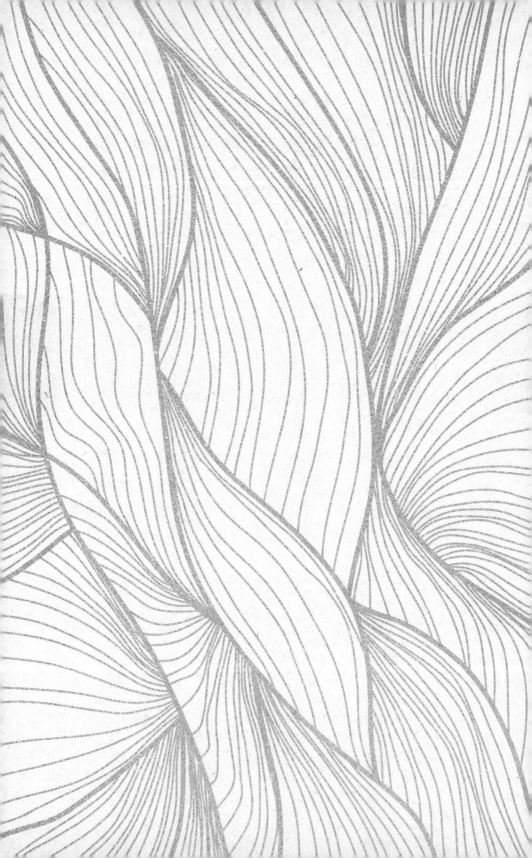

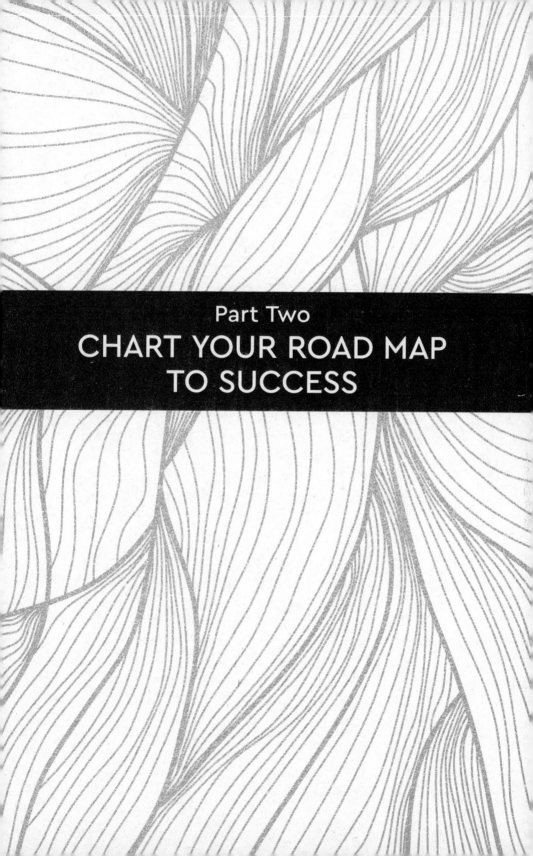

Part Two

CHART YOUR ROAD MAP TO SUCCESS

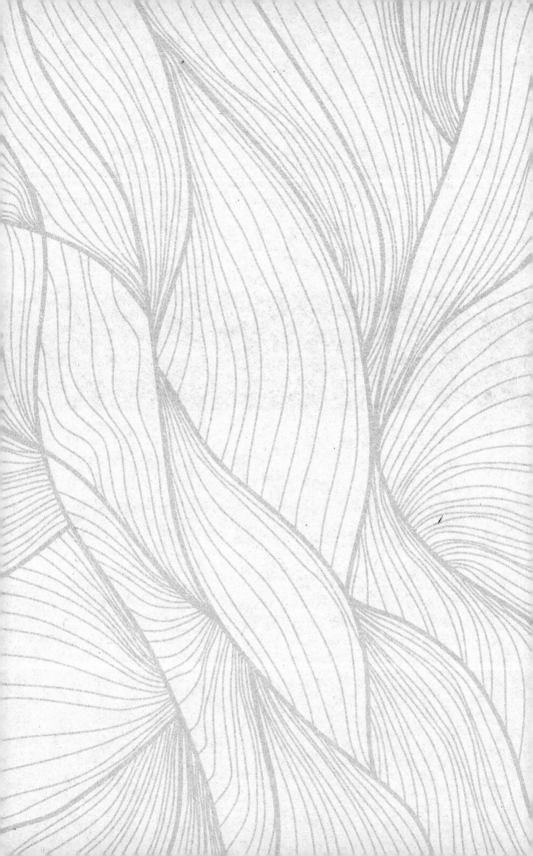

4.

~~~~~~~

Slam-Dunk Success with
Nutritional Science

B efore we dive into my action plans for success, I want to address one of the biggest obstacles many of us face when attempting to get healthier: how are we supposed to know which nutritional guidelines to follow when there's so much conflicting (mis)information? Examining clinically verified, publicly available data can help us avoid confusion and find a practical path toward healthier living.

The Lyon Protocol's nutritional strategies are a critical component of your road map to success. **Assembling accurate information that will help you stay focused on your objectives is a key part of developing a fail-proof plan.** To keep us motivated, it's crucial that we understand the true consequences of our choices, both positive and negative. This means tackling, head-on, any health-care biases we may have absorbed.

Since so much of the widely circulated nutritional "wisdom" is built upon a set of faulty premises, it's likely that the bulk of the "science" you've been exposed to needs a serious upgrade. Knowing *what to do* is only one part of this program. Another keystone is learning *how to think* about nutrition so you can bring a discerning eye to your daily choices and can vet any new health information that comes your way. The opportunity to help you correct any misconceptions is my greatest privilege. It's also a heavy lift that requires parsing some science and some history. But don't worry. I'll break down the information into bite-size pieces.

Modern dietary science is a relatively young discipline. Back in the early twentieth century, the study of human nutrition primarily consisted of chemists examining the protein, fat, and carbohydrate composition of foods. Not until 1926 did scientists isolate and identify the first vitamin. This kicked off five decades of research focused on preventing nutrient-deficiency diseases. More recently, focus shifted to nutrition's influence on chronic conditions such as cardiovascular disease, diabetes, obesity, and cancers, especially after 2000.[1] We're still living with the legacy of past priorities and findings—even some that more recent research has since dismissed.

I often wonder what it was like for the earliest nutritional scientists eager to share new information with the public. I imagine the process went much as it does today, with countless individuals chiming in with their own opinions, including "influencers" whose amplified voices can carry their messages the farthest. Part of my objective here in this chapter, within this very truncated version of the history, is to highlight how science reflects the perspectives of each historical moment. As part of helping you navigate the floods of food science information, I want to highlight how nutrition advice and cultural movements go hand in hand. I also want to teach you tricks for reading behind the headlines to evaluate the accuracy of any latest nutrition news, by presenting a primer on evidence quality.

THE BIRTH OF NUTRITION SCIENCE AND
DIETARY GUIDELINES

SPOILER ALERT: Our country's dietary guidelines were not designed with you in mind.

Instead of prioritizing optimal health for individuals, that is, YOU, nutritional recommendations have been influenced by political and policy considerations since the beginning.[2] Unpacking the history of these guidelines reveals the origins of the muddied waters of misinformation that have left so many of us over-fat, under-muscled, and wholly confused. Politics, social agendas, morality, and religion have always played a role in dietary choices, but did you know how significantly such external factors have affected nutrition science?

As a physician focused on facts and outcomes, I find it fascinating to examine the tremendous impact that extraneous political and social forces have had, over time, on what we feed ourselves. One fascinating example of the entanglements of diet and morality was the tremendous influence in the mid-1800s of a Presbyterian minister named Sylvester Graham (for whom the cracker was named), who's referred to as the "Father of Vegetarianism." Out of concern that both meat and alcohol promoted gluttony, harming individuals, families, and society, Graham called for a "simpler, plainer, and more natural diet" that excluded meats, white flour, condiments, and spirits in favor of consuming more fresh fruit and vegetables. Proclaiming that wholesome food made wholesome people,[3] Graham helped to launch one of America's first plant-based movements. The diet he prescribed was presented as an antidote to social, spiritual, and physical corruption. This movement away from animal protein toward carbohydrate consumption was further promoted by a follower of Graham named John Harvey Kellogg. Yes, *that* Kellogg, of the cereal brand, who created a "granola" cereal in 1878. I find it fascinating to consider the incredibly powerful influence these two men continue to have on the Standard American Diet (SAD) of today.

WARTIME CALCULATIONS

Religiosity isn't the only social force that has swayed American food-ways. War has always played a role as well. Pragmatic questions about how best to fuel a fighting force have steered the science and funded targeted research in significant and lasting ways. In 1917, President Woodrow Wilson established the US Food Administration to ensure adequate fare for World War I troops fighting overseas. Led by Herbert Hoover, who pioneered the slogan "Food will win the war," the agency worked to control the supply, distribution, and conservation of food, in part through the designation of certain days on the home front as meatless, sweetless, wheatless, and porkless.

Before World War II, scientists were still working to identify vitamins and minerals in food. Then suddenly, under the pressure of impending American involvement, the makeup of a healthy diet had geopolitical ramifications. During the Depression, economic hardship had led to low-protein diets and malnourishment in large portions of the American population. When the military struggled to find sufficient healthy troops for deployment, the government sought help from leading nutritional scientists and funded centers that would serve as the backbone for nutrition as a health discipline.

Once the US entered the war, food consumption was dictated by rationing, since most nutrient-dense food and protein were sent overseas.[4] Hoover issued warnings in January 1943 about the state of American meat supplies. He declared that "meats and fats are just as much munitions in this war as are tanks and aeroplanes,"[5] emphasizing the patriotism of abstaining at home to benefit the troops.

The next three decades saw expansion of nutritional research that significantly furthered understanding of food, physiology, and food processing—but from a particular vantage point and for the purposes of fulfilling a specific agenda: fortifying soldiers. The studies conducted then live on to this day. Their findings continue to underlie dietary guidelines affecting all of us, despite the research having been conducted primarily on young men rather than on women, children, or older adults. **Geared toward preventing deficiencies and focused explicitly on boosting short-term performance rather than optimizing long-term health, government-funded studies led to the development of dietary guidelines that still influence us today.**

Tracing nutrition trends over time grants new insights into the different forces steering the ship. Just think, four decades after wartime rationing limited access to much-sought-after meats and other animal products, individuals began to *self-impose* protein restrictions during the low-fat, low-cholesterol craze of the 1980s. This time, the shift was based not on rations or patriotism but on public pressure and misguided information. How is it that we've wound up demonizing the same high-quality proteins once recognized as so valuable that the home front must forgo them for the sake of the soldiers? And how has this progression led us to the plant-protein imitation "meat" craze of today?

Let's investigate . . .

To repeat, it's critical to recognize that the goal of government-funded nutritional guidelines was *never* to help individuals achieve exceptional health. Instead, setting forth *minimum* intake values was intended to prevent deficiencies. As we've seen, early studies focused on micronutrients—the vitamins and minerals that we need for survival—and rightly so. Micronutrient deficiencies are deadly in the short term.

Take the diseases scurvy, rickets, and beriberi. Each of these results from the lack of one specific nutrient. Scurvy, caused by vitamin C deficiency, for example, killed two million sailors between the sixteenth and eighteenth centuries before the Royal Navy and the US Navy started adding vitamin C to rations.[6]

Throughout history, answers to the question "What do we need to supply for these soldiers?" have continued to establish benchmarks for nutrition levels that subsequently get applied to all of us. Interestingly, today's mainstream dietary recommendations, to eat less protein and more grains, in some respects mimic the Great Depression diets that once left so many malnourished. Only today, this approach to food is

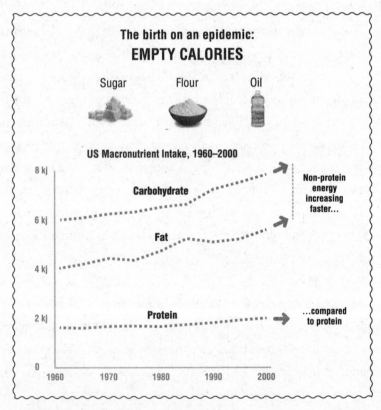

GRAPH CREDIT: Ted Naiman, MD

wrapped in a different narrative. Throughout history, meat has been cherished by humans. But over the last few decades, it has fallen from grace in favor of "unapologetically processed" plant-based "meats." Unfortunately, this has not resulted from new evidence and scientific rigors but more from industry, policy, and academic discourse.

Nutrition science has long been peppered with problems resulting from oversimplification, a focus on fat as the source of health issues, and failures to adapt to new scientific information. Neglecting the important role of protein in health and longevity has come with major consequences. Before I dig deeper into unpacking the politics and propaganda surrounding nutrition science, I want to arm you with tools to evaluate all the health advice flooding the media.

QUALITY OF EVIDENCE

High-quality discussion requires high-quality evidence. To keep you from getting swept up in the latest fitness frenzy, let's talk through what kinds of evidence should be informing your health decisions. Evaluating nutrition guidelines requires us to understand that not all the consumer-accessible information about the food we eat carries equal weight. Far too often, randomized controlled trials (RCTs) and other high-quality evidence get overlooked in favor of conclusions drawn from correlation rather than causation. One reason RCTs wind up getting deemphasized is that they often involve small numbers of participants. That's because it's difficult to control all aspects of a human life—unless subjects are living in a metabolic ward where the set conditions are far from everyday reality.

In a metabolic ward, an individual lives within a small, sealed chamber where a known composition of gas pumped into the space supplies the only air. The person breathing consumes oxygen and expels carbon dioxide. This gas exchange, monitored by sensors in the room, allows precise calculation of the energy expended. The ratio of oxygen to carbon dioxide can be used to determine whether an individual is burning primarily carbs or fat. To measure rates of protein oxidation, researchers analyze collected urine. Not exactly a regular daily routine, right?

Research challenges like these lead to the proliferation of "studies" reliant on low-quality evidence and to emotional responses and opinions getting mistaken for fact and pushed out to the public because they make great headlines. No wonder it's so difficult for consumers and laypeople to access quality information. This phenomenon is why I want to take some time to guide you through how to gauge the information that comes your way. Step one is to understand the hierarchy of evidence quality.

Here is the breakdown. The lowest quality of evidence consists of background information or expert opinions that lack corroboration. For example, if I tell you protein is ideal for weight loss because I have "seen" it work, don't believe me—at least, not until I present you with the evidence and explain the mechanisms through which the process functions. Without solid science to back up a statement, an expert can give nothing more than their opinion. (Fortunately, I'm deeply committed to rooting all my recommendations in high-quality, verifiable studies, and if I share an opinion based on clinical experience, I will say so!)

Next on the ladder of evidence quality comes the observational studies "rung." This evidence includes case studies and reports, cohort studies, and case-control studies, all of which observe people over time, or retroactively, without any intervention. Considered *weak* evidence because it can't prove causation, these types of findings *can* offer insights into concepts worthy of further inquiry. The key value of these approaches is to generate *hypotheses to be tested* using high-quality studies like RCTs.

While observational studies play a role in developing good science, they do not constitute good science in and of themselves. Because they rely on correlation without causation, they should not be used to make health claims. Despite that fact, the current health and nutrition landscape relies heavily on correlation data because these are readily available. With no requirement for actual intervention, researchers have far fewer variables to control. Case reports, meanwhile, constitute weak evidence simply because they're based on just one case.

Keep in mind that many strongly correlated factors may have absolutely no actual connection. Consider an absurd example. Over a ten-year period, the per capita consumption of margarine in the United States and the divorce rate in the state of Maine correlated at a level of 0.99 (the highest possible correlation being 1.00).[7] And yet, presumably, one did not cause the other. See the problem with this kind of thinking?

The gold standard of strong evidence comes from the RCT. Scientists use hypotheses generated from observational data and create an experimental setting where they can control for outside (confounding) variables. While observational studies cannot provide these benefits, RCTs allow for isolating the hypothesis to connect causes with effects.

Other criteria to consider when evaluating studies include sample sizes, exclusion criteria, and relative risk. The best health and nutrition data we have come from well-designed, reproducible RCT studies drawn from a large body of knowledge. Results from multiple RCT studies on a given topic can also be reviewed and analyzed in what is called a systematic review. While not as foolproof, given that the quality of the overall findings relies on the quality of each original RCT, systematic reviews can provide extremely valuable information. Statistical examination results in a meta-analysis, which is a valid, objective, and scientifically sound method of analyzing and combining different results.

By now, you might be asking, "What exactly am I supposed to do with all this evidence information?" **I have just given you the formula for distinguishing between sound science and hype. I've armed you with the tools necessary for evaluating data rather than simply accepting common nutritional narratives.**

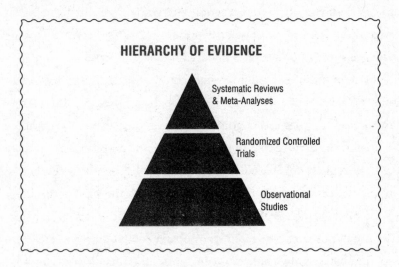

The next time some headline pops up on your Google feed, dig a little deeper. First, ask yourself: Is this news based on a study or opinion? If the information comes from a published, peer-reviewed paper, ask if the research was done on animals or humans. Next, look at the hierarchy of evidence pyramid to see where the study fits. If the findings result from research lower on the base of this pyramid, then you'll know to use a discerning eye while examining the information, rather than just accepting it at face value.

Before long, you'll notice that nearly all the information in the health and wellness space focused on extremes comes from low-quality data packaged with emotion. This is your first step toward unwrapping the information for yourself rather than relying on "experts" willing to discount data that doesn't fit their agenda.

■

Now that you understand the different types of data that get interpreted and applied to recommendations and policies, it might be a bit clearer how disagreements between parties can arise—particularly among people defending their own agendas. The reality is, from the moment the very first nutritional guidelines were ever issued, there were always other priorities and concerns at play.

I believe that individuals given access to clear, sound, and verifiable information can be trusted to make good, healthy choices. With that in mind, this chapter will help you:

1 Understand the facts that shift established paradigms, and

2 Engage with the transparent conversations necessary for true, lasting health and wellness.

THE PLAYERS

Who gives nutrition advice?

Why is dietary advice so confusing and often contradictory? Short answer: because the list of parties authorized to give us nutrition information reads like an alphabet soup. USDA, NIH, WHO, NAS-FNB. Compounding the issue is that all these agencies factor not just evidence-based nutrition science into their public policy recommendations but also food-industry priorities. Keep in mind the power that these standards hold, making them far more than just suggestions. The Dietary Guidelines provided by the USDA and the NIH establish US government public policy that impacts any facility receiving public funding. Schools, nursing homes, hospitals, prisons, day cares . . . all of these must design meals based on these guidelines. Meanwhile, the NAS-FNB (the National Academy of Sciences Food and Nutrition Board), which has no implementation authority, establishes Dietary Reference Intakes (DRIs) based strictly on science.

USDA or FTC? The Truth about Health Claims (and Restrictions)

Not only did US military research dollars spent on nutritional science prompt foundational dietary recommendations, but the funding also spurred major changes in food processing that gave packaged-food companies increased influence over which nutritional information reaches consumers. Because packaged foods and commodities are regulated under different agencies, the marketing dollars spent to promote packaged and processed foods far outscale those of commodity (agricultural) producers. In 2021, PepsiCo invested $1.96 billion in advertising in the US.[8] This staggering figure represents just one company in one country. Multiple behemoths flex their monetary muscle in a marketplace where the collective group of all commodities work to stretch their budget of $750 million. The major monetary imbalance of influence is clear.

What Are Commodities?

You've surely heard the campaign slogans "Beef. It's what's for dinner"; "Pork. The other white meat"; "Got milk?" Notice none of these mainstream campaigns advertises one specific supplier or brand. Instead, they reference a collective product. Messages such as these are government-sanctioned, producer-funded efforts to enhance the demand for farm commodities.[9] The term "commodity" refers to basic agricultural products such as soy, corn, wheat, coffee beans, sugar, palm oil, eggs, milk, fruits, vegetables, beef, cotton, and rubber.

A commodity is not a "brand." A brand (think Campbell's soup) has a company, budget, and professional team dedicated to developing creative marketing and communications programs to set it apart from competitors (say, Progresso soups). Now think about beef. While multiple brands are available, their products are still largely sold as beef, which can come from one rancher or another (as well as various other purveyors along the production chain). These producers lack the means to market their steak over another steak. So to compete in the marketplace, farmers and ranchers pool their money to promote and market whole categories of goods to consumers. The "checkoff" is a self-help program whereby producers pool their resources to collectively increase demand and awareness for products such as eggs, milk, and beef. The US Department of Agriculture (USDA) has oversight to ensure the checkoff programs are fair to all producers. The agency also restricts and regulates what health claims can be made to the public about these goods.

Commodity producers can say their products are part of a heathy diet, but they cannot say, for example, "Beef is a superior source of bioavailable zinc, iron, and protein." This difference illustrates a little-understood nuance between marketing/promotion abilities for consumer-packaged goods (CPGs) and commodities. The Nutrition Labeling and Education Act (NLEA) requires that CPGs have labels with standardized nutrition facts. But the USDA holds commodity communications to an even stricter level beyond the labeling rules. Commodities cannot compare their products with other foods— by citing the protein quality difference between beef and beans, for example—because that could be construed as disparaging beans.

While producers are permitted to provide the facts—for example, "Beef contains nine essential amino acids" or "Milk is good for your bones"—they cannot say the calcium in milk is more bioavailable than in almond milk. That's because commodities, marketed as a collective, cannot compete by making claims against one another. See the distinction?

Producers cannot add subjective, qualitative statements to marketing, such as "Beef is a better choice for helping to build and maintain your muscle because it contains all the essential amino acids," even though the statement is true.[10] Unlike those made by processed-food companies, every marketing statement—especially those related to health and nutrition—made by a commodity must undergo a strict scientific review as part of the checkoff program. One advantage of this rigorous vetting, for consumers, anyway, is that you can have increased confidence in commodity claims.

The standards for processed foods are far less precise, giving CPGs more leeway for hyperbole. Processed-food producers are not regulated by the USDA but instead fall under Federal Trade Commission (FTC) guidelines. They cannot claim a product will cure disease but *can* make a broad range of health claims—including claims *against* commodities, with statements such as "Eggs are bad for you," while their oat cereal is "heart-healthy." Meanwhile, egg producers have no mechanism to dispute false claims or financially support sustainable, evidence-based public education. Although sellers and producers of packaged foods are subject to FTC violations/lawsuits for making misleading statements, it is impossible for the FTC to sheriff all the crazy stuff out there. One powerful new force in the competition between processed and unprocessed foods is the plant-based "meat" companies. Food manufacturers like these employ sophisticated marketing techniques that can push limits and wind up spreading misleading information. So, from a marketing perspective, CPGs and commodities don't really compete on a level playing field.

As you can see, commodities end up like a mouse with the microphone trying to be heard over the small group of packaged-food companies that own and control most of the messaging. Suffice it to say that hidden influences, from market to military, have played key roles in the development of popular nutrition narratives. As a result, both doctors and laypeople unknowingly use misinformation that can lead to deadly decisions. The minimal nutritional information that physicians are taught in medical school is a by-product of agenda-based—instead of evidence-based—medicine. This trickles down to create wellness handcuffs for both doctors and their patients.

THE BENEFITS OF PROTEIN, UNDISPUTED

Energy, money, and attention are, of course, finite resources. Focusing on one area of the science (fat and cardiovascular disease, for example) at the expense of another (e.g., protein, which was largely ignored in nutrition science for quite some time) can leave us all with skewed information. Interestingly, despite being underrepresented and underrecognized, the benefits of protein have, unlike fat and carbs, long remained undisputed. Recommendations about carbohydrates have flip-flopped over the years. Different types of fat have been demonized and then redeemed. Meanwhile, protein hasn't been questioned so much as it's been left out of the conversation entirely.

Perhaps surprisingly, researchers' focus on fat wound up establishing protein as the most important and underappreciated macronutrient. Today's dietitians are trained that once they've determined a client's or patient's overall energy needs, **the first and most important nutrient to calculate into an individual's diet is protein. Only *after*** protein intake is established do they backfill the remaining calories with carbohydrates and fat.

Does this suggest that government guidelines are finally catching up to the centrality of protein? Since policy stipulates a five-year review schedule for nutritional recommendations, today's standards must be keeping pace with scientific progress, right? You guessed it: not so much. Despite protein's critical role in good health and longevity, the macronutrient was all but ignored in public health guidelines between 1980 and 2010. For the past three decades, protein recommendations have remained static—at a subthreshold level. This is a key point and a clear example of how consumers can get left in the dark on critical information that can significantly impact their health. The fact is, **despite the basic training that all dietitians receive, the current government guidelines first address *carbohydrates and fats* before allocating protein recommendations, as a percentage of energy in relation to these other macronutrients.** This is a significant flaw, with real consequences. Here's why.

The fewer calories you consume, the more these calories should come in the form of dietary protein. But because protein is an absolute requirement, it may be misleading to consider it as a percentage of calories. That's because, depending on your calorie consumption, you could wind up eating too little. Here's how this plays out. If we follow the guidelines recommending that protein make up 15 percent of caloric intake, a 70-kg adult consuming 2,500 kcal/day would get 93 grams of protein. However, that same individual on a lower-calorie diet at 1,400 kcal/day would consume only 52 grams of protein, which is too low for healthy muscle.

In chapter 5, we will dig even deeper into protein quantity, quality, and timing, but first, a quick preview is relevant to our discussion here.

Animal-based products provide high-quality, nutrient-dense sources of protein, which becomes especially important when you consider that we don't eat for protein, per se, but for amino acids. (Stay tuned for more on the exact ins and outs of eating for aminos.) You *can* get enough protein from plants, but this may not be an ideal strategy due to the carbohydrate and caloric load of plants, as well as nutrient density.

The recommended dietary allowance (RDA) for protein, which, as we've discussed, represents the *minimum* amount to prevent deficiency, hasn't changed for thirty years. All existing reliable science makes clear that today's recommended dietary allowances—for protein, in particular—are nowhere near optimal. The current RDA calls for 0.8 grams of protein per kilogram of body weight. I, meanwhile, recommend a baseline of 1.6 grams per kilogram, prioritizing the needs and wellness of the individual. (This recommendation is rooted in groundbreaking research on the leucine threshold necessary to trigger muscle-protein synthesis, which I'll discuss in detail on page 122.) My prescription, simply put, is that **every adult should consume at least 1 gram per pound of their ideal body weight each day. In particular, your first and last meals of the day should each contain a minimum of 30 grams of high-quality protein.** One source of food-policy pressure is the WHO, which aims to establish requirements that underdeveloped countries can meet. Like other nutritional guidelines, WHO recommendations are not about optimal health for individuals but are about economics and achieving minimum standards of health for the underprivileged. Efforts to make policies accessible to different countries across the world reflect attempts at standardization. Decisions to lower protein recommendations are not about health. To put it plainly, adopting policies concerned with global health would require lowering standards in the US, strictly for inclusivity's sake.

My advice is this: if you have the resources for optimal health, don't shortchange your well-being. We might live in a global food environment, but forgoing the flank steak will not deliver it across the globe to someone else's table. That's just not how things work. Instead, I urge you to consider the unintended consequences of lowering the quality of your diet. A huge increase in health problems and associated costs, perhaps? If we lower the quality of food we eat for the sake of some common denominator, something has to give. What's the trade-off? Even if you could offset the costs to both the body and the environment of prioritizing protein, it's critical to also consider the resulting price to be paid both physically and environmentally.

Contrary to the messaging many of us are getting today, a hearty steak as part of your diet is better for you than ultra-processed plant-based foods such as Twinkies, Lucky Charms, and Impossible Burgers. More than 12 million Americans have purged all meat from their diets, according to a recent Gallup survey.[11] And tens of millions more have slashed their consumption of steaks and burgers.[12] Based on USDA data, the US per capita consumption (pounds per person per year) of beef from 1970 to 2020 fell an annual average of 34 percent with no health or environmental benefits. Yet we still blame red meat for nearly all health problems. This terrifies me as a physician.

High-quality animal protein is the original superfood that plays a pivotal role in health. A recent study published in the *Journal of Nutrition* concluded that adults need to source 45 to 60 percent of their total proteins from animals to ensure sufficient levels of other nutrients.[13] If people keep shunning red meat in favor of low-quality plant-based foods, including cereals, breads, pastries, and pizzas, chronic disease rates will continue to skyrocket. It is well established that animal-based protein sources contain other vital nutrients such as iron, zinc, calcium and vitamin B_{12}. As people decrease animal-based proteins, they also impair the overall nutrient adequacy of their diets. When people eat less red meat, they typically fill up on highly processed convenience foods instead. The current American diet already consists of greater than 60 percent ultra-processed foods. Avoiding animal-based foods has already been associated with higher consumption of ultra-processed foods, largely in the form of commercial breads (refined and whole grain), ready-to-eat breakfast cereals, cakes, sweet snacks, pizza, french fries, soft drinks (sodas and fruit drinks), and ice cream.[14] These studies reflect the trend I've seen over my years in practice: when individuals cut back on animal-based foods, they don't compensate with plates of spinach but eat junk food instead. Another crucial point is this: the two most-consumed vegetables are potatoes and tomatoes. Nearly 70 percent of these potatoes are processed or frozen and eaten as french fries, mashed potatoes, or chips. Sixty percent of the tomatoes consumed are canned, often eaten as ketchup and pizza sauce.[15] Clearly, not all vegetarian or vegan diets have health benefits. Blanket advice to eat plant-based with an anti-animal spin deserves much of the blame for surging chronic disease rates.

SHIREEN'S STORY

I saw the damage of plant-based propaganda in the suffering of my twenty-five-year-old patient Shireen. Trying to "eat clean" to balance the effects of her fast-paced New York City life as she started her event planner career, Shireen ate a largely vegan diet consisting mostly of fruit in juices and smoothies. She exercised regularly but had incredible difficulty sustaining the energy to make it through her workouts. She was thin, with very low muscle mass, and struggled with regular episodes of low blood sugar. She had irregular menstrual periods and was losing her hair.

I helped Shireen transition slowly to the Lyon Protocol since she hadn't eaten animal products in almost a decade. We reduced her fructose intake and replaced it with protein shakes that were initially plant-based before moving gradually toward whey protein. Adding red meat to her diet just once a week led to astonishing transformations. Within three months, she'd become a new person. Her hair stopped falling out, and her periods became regular. Even her eye color changed and got clearer. In just twelve weeks, Shireen put on two pounds of muscle and lost nine pounds or 3.2 percent of body fat. Because of her age, she was able to get away with a bit lower protein amount than I typically recommend, but we still saw dramatic results. Shireen had been acting upon good intentions with bad information. Clear guidance and evidence-based intervention made all the difference.

MEAT MYTHS

Portrayed as unhealthy, unsustainable, and unethical, animal products have been demonized in recent decades, particularly in the urban West. It's remarkable how all-pervasive this messaging has become, despite the significant health benefits of consuming these nutrient-rich food sources. Did you know that eating less animal protein has been linked with an increase in waist size among women?[16] Far too often, people reducing their consumption of animal proteins replace them with carbs. Carbs from green vegetables such as kale or broccoli can be great for our health, but people tend to gravitate toward foods such as white bread, pasta, chips, and french fries, which offer little nutritional value. More than 40 percent of Americans' daily calories come from low-quality carbs, according to a Tufts University study of nearly 44,000 adults from 1999 to 2016.[17]

The trend toward plant-based foods is decades in the making. In the 1990s, nutritionists told Americans that fat was the root of all health problems. When SnackWell marketed its cookies as healthy "no-fat" alternatives, Americans ate so many that the brand surpassed Oreo in sales. Despite the "healthy" messaging, customers were consuming nearly the same number of calories as with traditional cookies—because fat had been replaced with sugar.

Today history is repeating itself, this time in a frenzy over plant-based fake "meat." Fast-food chains are rolling out plant-based alternatives like Burger King's "Impossible Whopper," which attempts to mimic a four-ounce real beef burger but contains less protein, five times as much sodium, more saturated fat, almost as many calories, and a long list of additives.[18] On no planet are these ultra-processed fake-meat products healthier or environmentally more friendly than real beef. Americans should think twice before replacing meat with plant-based foods. One significant advantage to consuming animal-sourced foods is the high bioavailability of nutrients that are much more difficult to obtain from plant foods alone. Animal products provide excellent sources of unique nutritional compounds that play critical roles in development, function, and survival of people at all ages.

A single four-ounce steak supplies 28 grams of protein—about half the minimum amount to prevent deficiency. (The current US RDA for men is 56 grams of protein daily, and 46 grams for women.) And our bodies process red meat more efficiently than proteins in soy or wheat. Various long-chain fatty acids (eicosapentaenoic acid and docosahexaenoic acid), minerals (zinc and iron), and vitamins (vitamin D and vitamin B_{12}) are either (nearly) absent or less bioavailable in plants, where antinutritional factors can make it harder for your body to absorb or use them.[19] In fact, red meat is even more nutrient-dense than chicken or fish. The combination of protein and all the other vitamins and minerals makes red meat a particularly bioavailable food that supports muscle health. While all animal-based proteins are highly bioavailable, red meat is one of the best dietary muscle meat sources of iron and B vitamins. Many organ meats have more vitamins and minerals, but the US diet does not typically include a lot of liver, heart, or kidney. As always, it's critical that we look at a food type as a whole rather than emphasizing just one aspect of its nutritional value. A quick look at the Food Pyramid reveals that the US has, in essence, been embracing plant-based diets for decades—and they've been killing us.

Here we can see how nutritional legacies carried forward to this day can lead to decisions based on misinformation. If only we could go back in time . . . Had we spent the last decades operating under the correct paradigm, we would have seen progress. We could have solved the problem. Dispelling the myths, misinformation, and misguided messaging that govern so many mainstream beliefs about health and nutrition is essential to cultivating a muscle-centric life plan.

BIAS AGAINST MEAT

The fat-focus "hangover" afflicting mainstream health recommendations is just one reason for the current bias against animal foods in the nutritional science community. Other complicating factors are the moral/ethical concerns about eating meat and/or dairy. This incredibly complex topic involves multiple considerations. The animal/plant divide has existed for ages. Midway through this century, vegetarian societies were founded amid a period of infrastructural changes in the food chain. These changes led to the loss of small family-owned farms and to the industrialization of livestock, which began to disconnect people from the processes of raising and harvesting animals for food.

As we've seen, the moral aspect of food choices is nothing new. For millennia, all the world's major religions have included dietary laws. More recently, in 1971, the book *Diet for a Small Planet* made a huge impact on society, shifting the purpose of a "good" diet to include both nutritional and environmental considerations.[20] This gave rise to new binaries such as artificial versus natural and animal versus plant.[21]

Increasingly, consumption of animal food products has been presented as unethical and harmful to both our health and the planet. Today some advocate a diet completely without, or with very low amounts of, these products. Some even call for the end of livestock farming in favor of processed-food companies that produce plant-based "meats" and "dairy." (The plant-based milk company Oatly cites as a "core objective" the goal "to promote plant-based nutrition over animal-based nutrition in every way possible.")[22] Food production does have a global link to the environment, and yes, climate change is real. But the truth is, **we are not going to eat our way out of climate change**.

Based on the current discourse, you might think the way to save the planet is to stop eating meat. Noise surrounding the heated topic of global warming can obscure and distort actionable steps. Recently, cattle have become a universal scapegoat. Environmental Protection Agency (EPA) scientists have quantified the impacts of livestock production in the US, which accounts for about 4.2 percent of all greenhouse-gas emissions (GHGE)—2.2 percent for beef cattle and 1.37 percent for dairy cattle.[23] In the grand scheme, these percentages are minimal. We can't blame cattle for the sins of fossil fuels.

ENVIRONMENTAL IMPACT BY THE NUMBERS

Highly publicized models designed to highlight the effect of eliminating all animals from our food production pipeline suggest this would reduce global GHGE by 28 percent.[24] However, the true numbers are much smaller. The GHGE from *all* agricultural practices in the USA only encompasses roughly 10 percent, with plant agriculture producing the majority.[25] Cutting animal agriculture would amount to only a 3 percent reduction in total GHGE nationally, or 0.5 percent globally.

These models also show that cutting animal products from the American diet would lead to increased deficiencies of essential nutrients (namely, amino acids and fatty acids) and increased overall calorie consumption as people try to meet minimal protein requirements.[26] As we've seen, these changes would only exacerbate the obesity and metabolic syndrome epidemics.

Another aspect often overshadowed in the current animal-versus-plant debate is how animal agriculture benefits sustainability initiatives. Consider that ruminant animals such as cows and sheep upcycle indigestible refuse from plant agriculture, converting it into meat enriched in essential amino acids and micronutrients including carnitine, creatine, zinc, heme iron, and B vitamins.[27]

These animals also play an indispensable role in the maintenance and restoration of topsoil and the carbon cycle.[28] Topsoil erosion resulting from modern industrial agricultural practices in the US has been estimated to contribute around 1 gigaton of carbon to GHGE,[29] which is around 20 percent of the total annual GHGE. Conscious incorporation of ruminant animals into land management also has the potential to reduce the agricultural requirements for synthetic nitrogen fertilizers, which are major contributors to emissions of the greenhouse gas nitrous oxide.[30]

Failure to recognize the positive contributions of ruminants to soil preservation and restoration would be a huge missed opportunity to significantly reduce our total GHGE over the next century. Prioritization of these objectives would not only reduce GHGE but also have an immense impact on water and air quality,[31] two other major areas of environmental concern.

Not only would eliminating animals from US agriculture have a nominal impact on overall GHGE, but removing animal products from the American diet would contribute to worsening of metabolic health in a society where more than 40 percent of adults are classified as obese.[32]

Over the years, I've seen patients struggle to make choices in alignment with what's right for their bodies, society, and the planet. These people often stay in a perpetual loop of frustration, caught up in the confusion of conflicting information. This is one of the dangers resulting from a single faction of scientists having a stronger foothold/ higher profile/larger influence on nutritional discourse—especially when sweeping public policies get driven by this influence. Today cracks are emerging in the stronghold, with growing appreciation of animal protein's importance.

"Protein quality is the one factor that the plant-based narrative can't defend very well," my mentor, Dr. Don Layman, has explained. "It's pure numbers, biologically proven." Arguing the superiority of a plant-centric diet based on epidemiology or distorted statistics on global warming is subjective and fallacious. These approaches produce a lot of interesting headlines, but no one can accurately argue with the fact that animal products provide higher-quality protein. It's time we stopped thinking of nutrition as either plant or animal but included both in our diet. Red meat is as old-school as it gets—the highest source of bioavailable proteins and amino acids—it's the OG of superfoods.

MINDSET RESET

SETTING (NOT GOALS BUT . . .) STANDARDS

Elite military operators abide by a set of principles that we can all learn from as we make real, lasting health improvements in our own lives. Take my patient Brian, for example, whose response to a life-altering accident epitomizes resilience and adaptability. A Texas farm boy built like a tree trunk—six feet tall and 260 pounds of muscle—Brian had served for fifteen years as an active-duty Navy SEAL. He was the guy they sent in to break down the doors. Despite multiple war deployments to some of the most dangerous places on earth, Brian had never gotten injured. Not until he returned home from overseas.

While riding his motorcycle at five miles per hour, he was struck by a teenager who'd been texting and driving. The bike got mangled, and Brian lost his leg from the knee down. In the months after, bone-crushing fatigue and pain led him to seek help from multiple physicians. Then he came to me. My Mama Bear type of doctor approach tends to work well with military guys. (They'll often put up with my prodding questions, without punching me in the face, ha ha!) As soon as I walked in the door, I headed for the sweet spot.

"Brian, I know this must be so hard for you. Here you are, this big, strong alpha dude with multiple deployments. You have had real life-and-death experiences, and yet you lost your leg to an irresponsible teenager. How are you feeling?" If he was going to complain, I had clearly set the stage.

His reply was "Well, ma'am, just what I had mentioned earlier. I'm pretty fatigued, and I'm having some phantom limb pain."

"I mean, how are you dealing with all THIS?"

He gave me this genuinely bewildered look and said, "Doc, what do you mean? Oh, you mean my leg? That was six months ago."

Get the picture? Brian had lost his leg just six months earlier, and yet he'd gotten past that and moved on to the next thing. Would you have moved on in six months? Most of us probably wouldn't have. As Viktor Frankl put it, pain is inevitable, but suffering is optional.[33]

The inner tape that dominates so many of us had largely been trained out of Brian. He didn't let his thoughts just "happen" to him; rather, he used his mind as a tool. Brian showed me that you can cultivate ridding yourself of harmful mental clutter. His proactive approach helped him adapt to the nutrition plan I created to protect him from skeletal muscle wasting due to his injury.

Brian focused on protein for recovery, eating whole, nutrient-dense foods. This helped limit any loss of muscle mass while we reworked his training program to meet his body's new realities. An example of someone taking full advantage of an exceptional mental framework, Brian never made excuses or said, "I can't." Recognizing that adopting a victim mindset would only pull him farther from his goals, he moved forward with his plan, geared toward muscle growth and protection, without getting caught up in a narrative that would hold him back.

Each of us processes information differently, based on our life experiences and how our brains are wired. No two humans are alike. This simple yet profound concept leads to highly individuated life outcomes.

CALLING THE SHOTS ON SELF-TALK

Instead of letting your inner monologue run the show, leverage it to your cause, coaxing your self-talk to encourage rather than disparage you. This can help push the lever of self-worth. In the beginning, that mental tape of inner commentary may be playing loudly, and it might be less than supportive. Once you learn to reframe the chatter and wrangle it to your cause, this voice can begin to help rather than hurt your progress.

What you say to yourself in those undercurrents will ultimately manifest in both how you feel about yourself and how you treat yourself. Self-worth becomes the director of your action. Think of self-worth as the luxurious interior of your dream house. Every day, you'll see those drapes you chose looking back at you. The same is true for the direct reflection of yourself that greets you daily.

Do you feel good about having a nice home? Do you deserve to have the home you want? Do you feel comfortable in that new body, with having exceptional health? What resources, time, and money are you willing to put into the house of your dreams? Self-worth determines how far you are willing to go in this department. How you feel about yourself determines your ability to control your behavior.

Results come when you prioritize your plan over any naysaying inner voice. It helps to get into the habit of noticing your thought patterns. Make a list. Name the different loops. And then you can start dealing with them. Here are some of my favorites:

- **Pessimist.** You catastrophize constantly, imagining the worst-case scenario on all fronts. If you are headed on a trip, you're sure there will be a massive pileup on your way to the airport. Standing in line at security, your head churns with images of the plane crashing. Time for your annual checkup? You're certain this will be the day they hand down a deadly diagnosis.

- **Frozen with Fear.** "Everything is so overwhelming; I am just going to do nothing." You hype up stress and hide behind the excuse of being overwhelmed. Your stress scale stays pinned to a rating of nine or ten. You cannot take your supplements because having to order them and lay them out for the week would be too taxing. Go to the gym? You can't do that, because all that equipment is so confusing, and you won't know what to do. Essentially, everything is impossible, providing a ready-made excuse for failure before you even begin.

- **Poor Me.** "I'll never get in shape. It's so much easier for everybody else." "I was born overweight, and my parents are not healthy." "My traumatic childhood keeps me leaning on food for emotional support." There are a million different versions of these constant comparisons to others. Thoughts like these run in a loop because the brain is good at repeating what it has practiced.

The three main results I see from negative thought patterns are depression, anxiety, and difficulties in physical health. Likely, one of your loops includes thoughts that could lead to any of these outcomes. Instead of letting that negative tape run circles around you, talk back to it. Once you have the list of your top loops, you'll know how to identify each one as it arises. Each time the voice on that tape pops up, address that loop directly. Transforming the monologue into a dialogue will help you take the reins in the conversation.

Take the Poor Me loop, for example. How should you respond to a voice that insists, "I'm so out of shape, I'll never get fit. Others have such an easier time of this"? The talk-back would include "Hey, I got this. I'm going to focus on the effort and executing like I'm supposed to." The goal is to reply with this every single time the Poor Me loop pops up. The easiest way to promote change is to remind yourself that your inner monologue does not define you, is not unique to you, and is not personal. In fact, you will always have self-talk of some kind, and some of it will likely always be annoying, negative, or downright insulting. The actions you take in response to the talk will determine who is in control, you or your mind. It's up to you to determine the steps that will accomplish your desired outcome and take them. And I'm here to help.

5.

~~~~~~~~~~

Protein: More Than Just
a Macronutrient

Roughly 60 percent of your body is water; half of the remaining 40 percent is protein. Your bones, ligaments, tendons, liver, brain, skin, and fingernails are all built from proteins. But this vital macronutrient is responsible for far more than just physical structures. Proteins are the master regulators of all that is happening in your body, controlling function in all tissues and organs, including muscle. They include enzymes—a class of proteins that catalyze all the chemical reactions within the body. Proteins also support energy production and cell-to-cell communication.

Proteins facilitate critical cellular functions, including balancing hormones, and serve as vital immune-system mediators. As we saw in chapter 2, antibodies that inactivate pathogens as part of your immune response are a type of protein, as are many hormones, including insulin. The thyroid hormones—which help regulate your blood glucose and metabolic rate and can impact growth hormone secretion and bone health—are made from amino acids provided by proteins. The brain uses protein-rich foods to produce neurotransmitters such as epinephrine (adrenaline), norepinephrine (noradrenaline), dopamine, and serotonin, which are essential to brain-cell communication. These chemicals are directly linked to neurological development, sleep, and mood regulation.

BENEFITS OF A PROTEIN-FORWARD DIET

- ➡ Balanced blood sugar
- ➡ Increased energy
- ➡ Mental clarity
- ➡ Decreased body fat
- ➡ Improved body composition
- ➡ Reduced cravings

By now, I hope you're clear on the vital roles that protein plays far beyond just building new muscle. There's no getting around its role in all the body's systems. **These functions make protein critical for longevity, metabolic function, and quality of life.** Scientific understanding of the importance of dietary protein has evolved greatly, yet the public remains largely uninformed. Moreover, as we've discussed, old news that's been debunked by the research remains so ingrained that even some physicians are still sharing outdated recommendations.

Now is your chance to finally gain clarity on the proper protein consumption that's necessary to run all these systems, based on the most current research. Designing your diet around the protein **quantity, quality,** and **distribution** that meet the needs for muscle optimization will provide abundant amino acids for all these other essential functions such as brain-cell communication, appetite regulation, and hormone production. With a protein-forward approach, all other nutritional priorities fall into place.

QUANTITY

First, let's talk about **quantity**. The current US RDA for protein is set at 0.8 grams per kilogram of body mass. For someone who weighs 150 pounds, this equates to just about 54 grams of protein per day. (The RDA of protein is 46 grams for women and 56 grams for men.) These numbers, based on old-school nitrogen balance methods developed for animal agriculture, grossly underestimate the actual requirements.[1]

In my practice, I find that most people are not getting enough protein, and many have no idea how much they aren't getting until they attempt to quantify it by tracking their intake. This is why your first step toward protein correction will involve keeping a food log and using a food scale to figure out exactly how much you're eating. (More on that in chapter 7.) Even if you are not currently protein-*deficient*, most likely you're not yet protein-*optimized* unless you've already been paying special attention to your protein quantity, quality, and distribution.

MYTH BUSTER

You may have heard the myth that higher-protein diets lead to kidney dysfunction. The data tell us otherwise.

A meta-analysis conducted by prominent protein researcher Stu Philips looked at higher-protein (HP) diets (≥ 1.5 g/kg body weight or ≥ 20% energy intake or ≥ 100 g/day) and their effects on kidney function. The indicator known as glomerular filtration rate (GFR) reflects any change in the efficiency of kidney function. When compared with normal- or lower-protein (≥ 5% less energy intake from protein/day) diets, HP diet interventions did not significantly elevate GFR relative to diets containing lower amounts of protein. Researchers concluded that HP intake does not negatively influence renal function in healthy adults.[2]

A systematic review of randomized controlled trials and epidemiologic studies conducted by Van Elswyk et al. found that HP intake (≥ 20% but < 35% of energy or ≥ 10% higher than a comparison intake) had little to no effect on blood markers of kidney function (e.g., blood pressure) when compared with groups following US RDA recommendations (0.8 g/kg or 10–15% of energy).[3]

WHY YOU SHOULDN'T IGNORE PROTEIN...

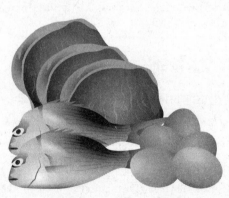

- Essential for cellular functions

- Influences metabolism

- Needed to build physical structures

- Impacts sleep and mood

- Needed for brain, bones, ligaments, tendons, liver, skin, and fingernails

PREVENTING MUSCLE AND TISSUE BREAKDOWN

All the tissues in your body are proteins. Over the course of a single year, nearly every one of these proteins gets replaced. It's mission-critical to ensure that you have sufficient and proper nutrients to meet, and exceed, these requirements. A body trying to make do with a low-protein diet will prioritize the survival of the liver, heart, brain, kidney, and gastrointestinal tract. Given the body's constant rebuild and repair cycles, these organs have high amino-acid demands, and your body will always work to take care of your organs first. Eating only enough protein to fuel these essential functions will leave your body lacking sufficient amino-acid supply to support skeletal-muscle growth and repair. By eating for muscle health, on the other hand, you will simultaneously meet all your primary biological needs while also optimizing for body composition.

Your body is counting on you to provide the ingredients necessary to supply its capacity to repair and rebuild. What exactly *are* those ingredients? It turns out, what we categorize as dietary protein includes a whole arsenal of specific amino acids.

PROTEIN QUALITY: AMINO ACIDS

We talk about protein as a single macronutrient, but it's just the delivery system for twenty different individual amino acids, which play dual roles: protein synthesis and the creation of new biomolecules and/or metabolic signals. This means all amino acids (AAs) have two primary purposes:

- Supporting the body's physical structure.
- Supporting physiological functions such as neurotransmitter and antioxidant production and protein synthesis.

It's important to grasp that we don't eat for protein, per se, but for AAs. Dietary protein is simply the vehicle. Protein's characterization as a single unit is one common roadblock to achieving a balanced dose of AAs. This means that **eating for protein quality requires adequate consumption of the individual AAs our bodies can't make** on their own. Check out the label on a food you eat regularly. See how macronutrients like carbohydrates are broken down into sugar, fiber, and total carbohydrates? Notice how fat is also differentiated into subtypes: saturated, trans fats, and cholesterol. Now find protein. Misleadingly, it's listed as just, well . . . protein.

But not all protein is created equal. Different protein sources do not have the same AA composition, and different combinations of the twenty AAs have unique properties and roles in the body. This is entirely overlooked in food-packaging requirements. Even the RDA doesn't recognize the meal requirements of different AAs. No wonder so many of us aren't taking in the quality proteins our bodies need.

There are twenty AAs, nine of which are designated "essential," which means they must be obtained through diet or supplementation because the body can't make them independently. We need to consume these in specific amounts to stimulate protein synthesis. When it comes to calculating our dietary protein intake, the real task is ensuring a proper balance of AAs absorbed through different food sources. This ensures that we have sufficient building blocks to fuel all the body systems I mentioned above, along with optimizing muscle-tissue maintenance and development.

We need three different types of AAs to maintain overall health:

- **Nonessential amino acids.** Your body produces these on its own, *if* you consume adequate total protein.

- **Conditionally essential amino acids.** In times of injury or illness, your body cannot make enough of these and relies on dietary sources.
- **Essential amino acids.** These come directly from your diet. Although they're called essential, even the aminos in this category are not *equally* essential. That's because it's harder to attain adequate amounts of certain AAs—such as leucine, methionine, and lysine—without consuming animal foods.

We'll delve more deeply into the essential aminos in a bit, but first, here's a list of the eleven "nonessentials":

- Alanine
- Arginine
- Asparagine
- Aspartatic acid
- Cysteine
- Glutamic acid
- Glutamine
- Glycine
- Proline
- Serine
- Tyrosine

In case you thought this could be simple, it's time for me to share that some of these nonessentials sometimes become essential. This gives them the honor of occupying a spot within the provisional category of *conditionally* essential AAs. Under normal conditions, the body can make these. But health challenges and increased metabolic demand

can leave the body unable to meet the physiological demands of production. Infection, surgeries, cancer, gastrointestinal issues, stress, and
intense prolonged physical activity can sometimes leave you short on:

- Arginine
- Cysteine
- Glutamine
- Glycine
- Proline
- Serine
- Tyrosine

Whenever your body can't keep up with production of these conditionally essential AAs, it's necessary to include them in your diet.

Let's look at glutamine, for example. The most abundant of all AAs,
glutamine is an incredibly versatile member of the conditionally essential
family that plays a pivotal role in maintaining the function of several
organ systems including the gastrointestinal tract, kidney, liver, and
heart, as well as neurons, and providing fuel for rapidly dividing cells.
Some of these quick-turnover cells include lymphocytes in the immune
system and enterocytes in the intestinal lining. As such, glutamine is
critical for both immune health and maintaining gut-barrier function.
More than 70 percent of circulating glutamine is derived from skeletal
muscle. Because branched-chain amino acids (BCAAs) are the only
AAs metabolized in skeletal muscles, the best way to increase glutamine
production in the body is by taking in an abundance of BCAAs. These
are naturally found in high-quality (aka animal-source) proteins and
act as a precursor for glutamine.

ESSENTIAL AMINO ACIDS

Now let's talk through the science of essential AAs. Don't worry. I won't put you through a biochemistry lesson on the unique characteristics of each of the nine aminos, but I do want to run through a few of the distinguishing features of these AAs that our bodies were designed to find in our environment rather than making them ourselves. These are the aminos we eat for.

ESSENTIAL AMINO ACIDS: PVT TIM HALL

If you *do* want to commit to memory the names of the nine unique essential amino acids, the mnemonic PVT TIM HALL can help.

- ◼ Phenylalanine
- ◼ Valine
- ◼ Threonine
- ◼ Tryptophan
- ◼ Isoleucine
- ◼ Methionine
- ◼ Histidine
- ◼ Lysine
- ◼ Leucine

It's pretty amazing, when you think about it, that all of our proteins are made up of only twenty AAs, some of which the body can make and others that must be taken in through food. For optimal health, some essential AAs must be eaten in specific doses (e.g., leucine).

Although each essential AA plays an important role in bodily function, three are uniquely important in characterizing food quality:

leucine, lysine, and methionine. These work best when consumed to-gether, and of these three, leucine is the most important for muscle health. Earlier, I described muscle-protein synthesis (MPS) and how consuming sufficient protein is necessary to stimulate this critical re-sponse. Now it's time to walk you through the science of the mamma-lian target of rapamycin (mTOR) mechanism, discovered in the 1990s by my mentor Dr. Layman. The crux of this breakthrough is the binary nature of mTOR's effect on MPS. Simply put, the dose of protein you eat in a single meal is either sufficient to trigger MPS or it isn't. Any diet that fails to meet this threshold is missing a key component to-ward the optimization of muscle and metabolic health.

The mTOR mechanism relies on leucine, a BCAA that, ingested at a particular dose per meal, fires up muscle tissue's protein-synthesis machinery. Leucine specifically activates a component of the mTOR signal complex, which plays a vital role in initiating and sustaining protein synthesis within cells. Think of leucine as the key you turn (or the button you push) in your car to fire up the engine. mTOR is the engine, and all the AAs your body has available supply the fuel. This whole system powers protein synthesis. While the mTOR mechanism is binary—either triggering MPS or not—this system is nuanced.

One major determinant of the mTOR threshold is age. When you are young and growing, mTOR is regulated by hormones (insu-lin, growth hormone, IGF-1), but as you age, skeletal muscle becomes "anabolically resistant." This means our bodies become less responsive to hormones and more sensitive to diet quality and the AA leucine.

PROTEIN NEEDS OVER TIME

Protein is the only macronutrient requiring age-based shifts in quan-tity and quality over time. While no carbohydrates are considered es-sential, your body's needs for essential AAs differ throughout your life span. Prescribing specific protein dosages to improve muscle health in your changing body is the peak of food-as-medicine. Leucine is a key driver of long-term positive physiological changes.

Because they are younger, children can reach the mTOR threshold with just 5 to 10 grams of protein. Some data suggest that active, healthy people in their twenties, potentially into their thirties, can get a robust MPS response from consuming just 1.7 grams of leucine at a given meal (although a higher range is likely better).[4] Several studies on older adults have shown that older people can experience a "restorative" effect on MPS from consuming at least 2.5 grams of leucine per meal. **That restorative level requires a minimum of 30 grams of high-quality protein at each meal.** To reach the leucine threshold by eating only plants, however, you would need to eat 35 to 45 percent more plant protein (depending on the source), which, of course, means consuming significantly more calories.

The potential for MPS restoration is significant here, especially from the perspective of early intervention. As we now know, aging begins in our thirties and forties, even if it goes largely unseen. MPS restoration evidence indicates that steps we take early on cannot only *protect* muscle tissue but even *restore* it. This finding demonstrates the urgency of learning about and implementing appropriate protein dosing as early as possible. Plus, check out this bonus: studies show that adding leucine-rich protein to meals not only triggers MPS but also helps stabilize your blood-glucose levels.

Most Americans today consume far less than ideal levels of leucine. Only about 25 percent of women ages fifty-one to seventy and just 10 percent of men in that age range were consuming the RDA, according to the National Health and Nutrition Examination Survey (NHANES) data. By age seventy-one and up, only half of women and about 30 percent of men reached RDA protein levels, according to

Berner et al.[5] These small percentages show just how few people older than fifty are consuming anywhere near enough protein to meet minimum muscle requirements. Although the science shows that **anyone who's older or under stress should consume roughly double the current protein RDA,** many people are not even *reaching* the minimum daily intake for protein, never mind doubling it. This is something we absolutely can, and must, correct.

Remember, RDA guidelines are based on a deficiency model, spelling out the *minimum requirements to keep you alive.* These indicate the lowest-level requirements needed to facilitate basic tissue repair but not much more. The RDA numbers also don't account for active lifestyles or the goal of protecting muscle and longevity as we age. For a better standard of measurement, I suggest you follow the **Lyon RDA.** Based on thirty years of scientific literature and Dr. Layman's discovery of the leucine threshold, **I recommend that adults consume 30 to 50 grams of high-quality protein** *at each primary meal.* Does that sound like a lot? Don't worry, I'll show you exactly how to make it happen. Remember, our goal here is not short-term survival (represented by the RDA) but long-term thriving (made possible by the Lyon RDA). Knowledge is power. Staying informed and educated will empower you to make the best decisions to live a long, strong, and healthy life.

QUALITY AFFECTS QUANTITY

It should be clear now why optimal health requires paying attention to the AA compositions of different foods. The proteins in beans or quinoa, for example, contain significantly different AA profiles from those of beef or chicken. If you choose lower-quality protein sources, you will need to consume greater quantities or find supplemental options. By and large, animal proteins, which contain the highest quantities of essential AAs, will serve you best in supplying the aminos critical for sustaining the body's protein-reliant systems—including muscle. It's not impossible to get these through eating an ovo-lacto vegetarian diet rich in dairy and eggs. It's not even impossible to get these in a vegan diet, although your options will be limited, and you might need supplements to prevent a deficiency.

Food per 1 oz	Methionine (grams)	Leucine (grams)	Lysine (grams)
Ground Turkey	0.140	0.385	0.455
Beef (top round)	0.260	0.793	0.843
Chicken Breast (skinless)	0.179	0.485	0.549
Tuna (yellowfin)	0.194	0.532	0.601
Pork Chop (lean)	0.189	0.584	0.635
Extra-Firm Tofu	0.350	0.210	0.182
Low-Fat Ricotta	0.800	0.346	0.379
Brazil Nuts	0.282	0.323	0.138
White Beans (large)	0.980	0.522	0.449
Navy Beans	0.270	0.179	0.148
Large Egg	0.106	0.305	0.256
Tempeh	0.490	0.400	0.254

For more foods, go to the USDA's website and search for leucine.

All this talk about essential AAs . . . but WHERE can you find them? The graphic on the following page shows AA overlaps among various foods. Listed at the intersection are foods rich in all three of these critical AAs, referred to as limiting AAs. You'll notice animal sources are the highest in these particular AAs.

Let's look back at our food label again. As you can see by the complex AA profiles of different proteins, the grams of protein listed for one food are not equivalent to the grams listed for another. In

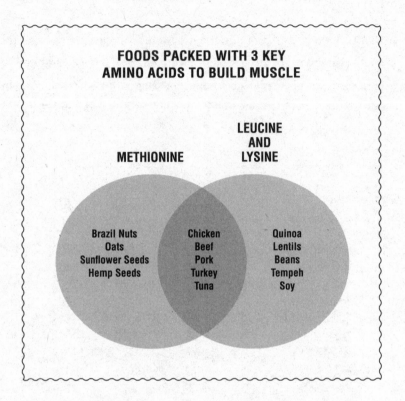

FOODS PACKED WITH 3 KEY
AMINO ACIDS TO BUILD MUSCLE

LEUCINE
AND
LYSINE

METHIONINE

Brazil Nuts
Oats
Sunflower Seeds
Hemp Seeds

Chicken
Beef
Pork
Turkey
Tuna

Quinoa
Lentils
Beans
Tempeh
Soy

other words, 6 grams of hemp protein does not equal the 6 grams of protein in an egg. Unfortunately, today's labels don't stratify foods based on protein quality or your body's ability to assimilate the protein you consume.

But fear not! I will teach you how to decipher labels, intentionally group AAs for optimal protein intake, and design nutritional strategies to ensure that you consume sufficient high-quality protein, properly dosed throughout your day.

COMPLETE VERSUS COMPLEMENTARY PROTEINS

Perhaps you've heard the term "incomplete protein" used to describe foods that are missing, or contain limited quantities of, one or more of the essential AAs in amounts necessary for human health. Legumes are a prime example. While they contain lysine, threonine, and tryptophan, legumes lack methionine. Grains, meanwhile, contain methionine but provide limited lysine and often limited threonine or tryptophan. Combined, legumes and grains supply a mixture of AAs of higher quality than either one alone. Such combinations are said to supply **complementary proteins** which, together, provide a full AA profile. Still, these mixtures are not as high in quality as the protein in meat, milk, eggs, or fish, given that the quantity of aminos they contain still may not be sufficient for protein optimization. Furthermore, combinations such as grains and legumes result in heightened carbohydrate intake that can result in excess calories for the average sedentary adult.

Protein protocols have been plagued with a tremendous amount of confusion that has major implications for overall health. Even people trying their best to eat healthy foods can fall into the trap of a low-protein

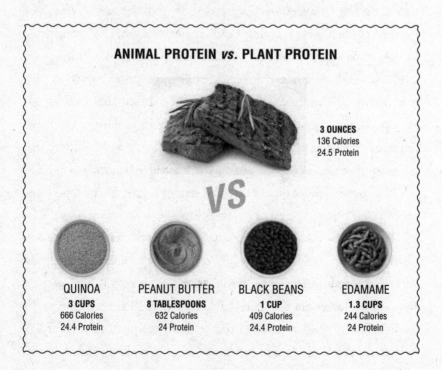

ANIMAL PROTEIN *vs.* PLANT PROTEIN

3 OUNCES
136 Calories
24.5 Protein

VS

QUINOA	PEANUT BUTTER	BLACK BEANS	EDAMAME
3 CUPS	**8 TABLESPOONS**	**1 CUP**	**1.3 CUPS**
666 Calories	632 Calories	409 Calories	244 Calories
24.4 Protein	24 Protein	24.4 Protein	24 Protein

diet that's impairing their ability to live their best life. Take Shanti, for example. A smart and health-literate professional in her late thirties, she came to me with dark circles under her eyes, emanating exhaustion. She wore baggy clothes and sat with her shoulders hunched over, her body language speaking volumes. Rarely do I meet a patient and worry that I might not be able to help them. Shanti was an exception. She felt sad and hopeless, weighed down by an overload of contradictory and confusing health and wellness information. Her defeated sense of herself and her health concerned me. Was she strong enough to improve her well-being? We discussed all that she'd been trying to do to improve her health. It quicky became clear that her macros were deeply out of balance.

Under treatment for chronic hypothyroidism, Shanti carried a few extra pounds but had no major weight challenges. The gap in her well-ness came from a misguided interpretation of the dietary advice she'd been given. She'd been trying her best to make what she considered healthy choices, carrying around food with her to keep within her or-ganic, whole-food goals. If it was a whole-food source robust in phy-tonutrients, vitamins, and minerals, Shanti was all about it. She ate rice and beans, veggies with quinoa, smoothies and shakes, and sweet potatoes. She had cut out red meat, consumed very little fish or dairy, but would eat the occasional egg. Shanti's unbalanced, carb-heavy diet left her anemic, short on energy, and struggling with low mood and overall well-being.

Reducing her carbs and increasing her protein dramatically improved Shanti's iron levels and her energy. But the most striking change I saw was in who she became as a person. Turning her diet around granted her a sense of freedom she'd never had before. Feeling better physically helped lift her mood. She used her newfound energy to seize control of her health, building strength inside and out. She no longer felt defeated.

VEGETARIAN DIETS

On average, vegetarians consume approximately 65 grams of plant-based protein a day, but this amount is far too low, especially given the quality of the amino acids consumed. While available evidence does not currently support recommending a protein requirement specific to people who consume only plant proteins, I expect this oversight will be corrected in the coming years— especially if we are focusing on whole-food diets rather than relying solely on augmenting protein status with protein powders.

Protein winds up being the most controversial macronutrient because animals have a face. But if optimal health and fat loss are our goals, we should put aside biases against these food sources. Extensive research shows that the highest-quality proteins come from animal sources, including meats—typically from gravity-bearing animals such as chicken, turkey, beef, bison, and lamb. Also helpful are eggs, dairy, and fish. In addition to having optimally balanced AA profiles, animal-based products are superior in calorie-for-calorie nutrient density. Moreover, their core nutrients are more bioavailable relative to plant foods.

PROTEIN POWER MOVES

- Eat your protein first. This will make sure you take in the AAs that drive MPS, and it will help you feel full sooner.
- Before you attend an event offering unhealthy food, drink a 20-gram protein shake.
- Replace salty, crunchy snack foods with Carnivore Crisps or other protein chips.
- Balance a low-protein meal by throwing a packet of AAs into your water. This can help activate your muscle metabolism and lower a spike in blood sugar.[6]

BEEF GIVES YOUR BODY...

...more of the nutrients you need. A 3-ounce serving of lean beef
provides the following nutrients in about 150 calories:

DV	Nutrient
8% DV	Calories
48% DV	Protein
48% DV	B_{12}
40% DV	Selenium
36% DV	Zinc
26% DV	Niacin
22% DV	B_6
19% DV	Phosphorus
16% DV	Choline
12% DV	Iron
10% DV	Riboflavin

BEEF BENEFITS

- Beef is a mighty nutritional powerhouse in a small package. Just one 3-ounce serving of cooked beef gives you ten essential nutrients.
- Protein helps preserve and build muscle.
- Vitamins B_6 and B_{12} help maintain brain function.
- Selenium helps protect cells from damage.
- Zinc helps maintain a healthy immune system.
- Niacin supports your energy levels and metabolism.
- Phosphorus helps build bones and teeth.
- Iron helps your body use oxygen.
- Taurine, carnosine, anserine, and creatine, absent from plants, are particularly abundant in beef.

MORE BENEFICIAL NUTRIENTS IN BEEF

■ Taurine, a non-proteinogenic AA that's essential for children (particularly preterm infants) and conditionally essential for adults, aids formation of bile salts that help eliminate cholesterol and absorb dietary lipids and vitamins. It also serves as a major antioxidant and has anti-inflammatory effects.

■ Carnosine reduces the formation of reactive lipid species and augments the restoration of glutathione blood levels.

■ Creatine is essential for energy metabolism in the brain and skeletal muscle. It has also been used to improve cognitive function and reduce the chronic effects of traumatic brain injuries.

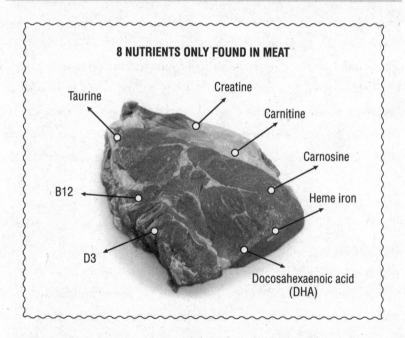

8 NUTRIENTS ONLY FOUND IN MEAT

Taurine

Creatine

Carnitine

Carnosine

B12

Heme iron

D3

Docosahexaenoic acid (DHA)

PROTEIN DISTRIBUTION TO MAXIMIZE MPS

We've discussed how the impacts of protein quality and quantity are deeply intertwined. The distribution or the timing of your protein consumption throughout the day makes a big difference too. Evidence suggests that typical American eating patterns set us up for poor muscle size and health throughout our lives. For instance, wolfing down a bowl of cereal or grabbing a bagel on your way out the door does not constitute the protein-packed breakfast needed to fire up your metabolism. Even people who eat an egg with toast or a small yogurt and fruit aren't taking in enough aminos to trigger MPS. Then, say your lunch consists of a small turkey sandwich or a salad, and dinner ends the day with a large steak and potatoes, fish and some veggies, or maybe some pasta. As you can see in the chart, this pattern will set you up for unbalanced protein distribution, which comes with consequences.

The costs of this imbalance over a lifetime wind up being significant. Not only do individual low-protein meals fail to adequately stimulate the body's capacity for protein synthesis (as discussed above), but these eating patterns can wind up establishing lifelong habits that serve us poorly. Over time, we find ourselves gaining body fat and losing muscle while becoming weaker and more fatigued. This damage gets compounded as our hormonal milieu changes over the years—when we fail to alter our dietary choices as hormone levels decline, we are left in an anabolic deficit.

Here's the good news: once you understand how to use food as medicine, the decisions you make can pivot you toward living your best life, both physically and mentally. Although some say total daily protein is most important, the literature suggests that distributing protein throughout the day is the optimal strategy for building and maintaining muscle. In my clinical practice, I've found that proper protein distribution throughout each day also increases compliance over the long term.

I've explained that my general recommendation to optimize MPS for most adults is to eat at least 30 grams of high-quality protein at each of three daily meals. But my specific recommendations for *you* depend on *your* specific goals. Are you trying to gain muscle? Then,

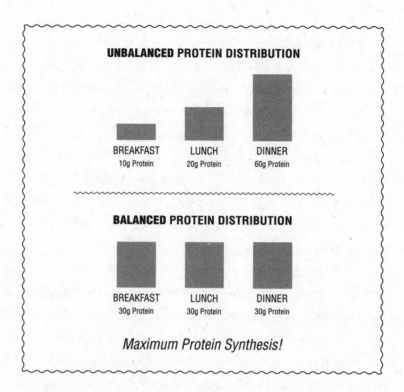

UNBALANCED PROTEIN DISTRIBUTION

BREAKFAST
10g Protein

LUNCH
20g Protein

DINNER
60g Protein

BALANCED PROTEIN DISTRIBUTION

BREAKFAST
30g Protein

LUNCH
30g Protein

DINNER
30g Protein

Maximum Protein Synthesis!

depending on your target daily total, you can increase your protein intake to four, five, or even six times a day. It's more effective to increase your total number of meals than to eat more protein at a single meal. For example, if your protein goal is 200 grams a day, and you've already planned three meals containing at least 40 grams of protein each, you should add an extra meal.

MEAL TIMING: BREAKFASTS AND DINNERS OF CHAMPIONS

When it comes to making muscle, breakfast is by far the most important meal. By breakfast, I mean your first meal of the day, whenever that is. A robust dose of protein, first thing, will set you up for metabolic optimization, priming your body by stimulating muscle growth, reducing hunger, and supplying you with an AA dose to use for other biological processes.

The second most important meal is the last one before your overnight fast. Choosing foods that provide your body with sufficient AAs
to generate glucose can help stabilize blood sugar through the night
and prep you for the morning. The International Sports Nutrition Society recommends pre-sleep casein protein intake of 30 to 40 grams
to fuel increased overnight MPS and increase metabolic rate without
negatively influencing rates of fat burning during sleep.[7]

A third pinnacle of protein timing is particularly helpful for people who are older, obese, or otherwise facing metabolic challenges
involving unhealthy muscle tissue. **Dosing protein after a bout of exercise, especially resistance exercise, promotes MPS.** Skeletal muscle
contractions result in increased blood flow, leaving the muscle tissue
primed to take in nutrients. (If you are new to exercise, trying to lose
weight, or recovering from an illness, then having protein after a workout is helpful for muscle responsiveness. I recommend a shake with
20 grams of whey protein.) In essence, prioritizing protein during this
period lowers the anabolic resistance of muscle tissue, allowing you to
get away with less dietary protein when it is combined with exercise.

PROTEIN'S SUPERPOWERS: THERMOGENESIS
AND SATIETY

Here's another advantage to eating more protein: satiety, that is, feeling
fuller for longer. Clinical trials comparing energy-balanced diets indicate that higher-protein diets are more satiating.[8] By consuming enough
protein throughout your day, you will be less likely to overeat. Think of
protein as the dietary means for augmenting your nutritional willpower.

Eating protein reduces feelings of hunger, which helps with fat loss
by facilitating adherence to a caloric deficit. Studies have also shown
that increased dietary protein, provided at breakfast, lunch, and dinner,
helps people feel both immediate and sustained fullness. This effect is

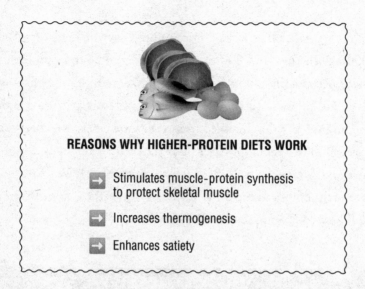

REASONS WHY HIGHER-PROTEIN DIETS WORK

→ Stimulates muscle-protein synthesis to protect skeletal muscle

→ Increases thermogenesis

→ Enhances satiety

produced by increased concentrations of plasma peptide YY (PYY), a gut hormone that drives fullness, as well as reduced levels of ghrelin, which drives hunger.[9] It turns out humans and many other animal species exhibit protein prioritization, meaning they will continue to eat until they have taken in an adequate quantity of protein, even if they must significantly overeat nonprotein energy (i.e., carbs and fat) to get there. Keep the protein percentage of your diet high, and you will tend to automatically eat less overall. Due to the thermic effect of food, you'll also burn more of the calories you do consume.

Let's break that down. Digesting, absorbing, and metabolizing macronutrients take energy, right? This energy requirement is called thermogenesis. So the thermogenesis of protein is the energy it takes for the body to process and use the protein you've taken in. Because of AAs' chemical structures and their fates within your body, it takes more energy to metabolize protein than carbs or fat. While traditionally calories from protein are calculated as 4 kcal/g, which produces the numbers on the back of your food labels, the digestion and assimilation of protein *increase* energy expenditure by 20 to 35 percent of protein's net caloric intake. For example, say you're maintaining a 2,000-calorie diet, and 800 of those calories come from protein; the digestion and assimilation of that protein will result in the burning of 160 to 240 calories. This is like consuming 20 to 35 percent less than the total protein calories tallied from your food labels. In other words, if you eat more protein, you kick-start your body's metabolic machine, and it's as if you've eaten less food overall! But now that we finally know how much protein to eat, what do we do about those confusing carb and flighty fat recommendations?

MINDSET RESET

IT'S JUST ANOTHER MEAL

Consistently choosing the foods our bodies need for balanced nutrition can be challenging for people—particularly when it comes to picking protein over carbs. Cultural narratives often get in our way. We tell ourselves stories that amp up the importance of each meal—treating it like it's our last. Consider the emotional weight we invest in a birthday meal, or Thanksgiving dinner, or a date night out. We often get wrapped up in anticipation of the food as the big event, building it up in our minds. But ask yourself: How often does the meal end up as good as you've made it out to be? Does that disappointment end up driving you to eat more or even to create another cheat-meal opportunity, all in search of culinary bliss? This is where nurturing a neutral mindset is key.

Rather than hyping up the food, revel in the experience and quality time. When your mind gets flooded with all the stories surrounding the meal, neutralize them. Remain steady. If you can talk yourself into how great something is, you can talk yourself out of it. This takes practice. Remember: it's not an emotional investment; it's just another meal.

Many mechanisms drive our desire to eat, including the dopamine-reward pathway. For me, learning about my own biology and beginning to understand my own areas of weakness brought huge relief. Finally, I began to grasp the conditions that pushed me off my nutrition plan and down a spiral of poor eating habits. I began to notice patterns. My vulnerable moments often arose right after I experienced the "high" of acing a test or giving a great talk. Right at that high point, I could feel cravings kick in, urging me to reach for foods outside my plan to keep that good feeling going.

Here's the hack for dealing with these kinds of cravings: Peer into your crystal ball and anticipate the future. Over time I learned that preparing myself ahead of time for these emotional swings helped me maintain equanimity—that neutral mental framework. Mitigating the emotional upswings helped me quell my cravings by harnessing the dopamine drive. Referred to as "the molecule of more," dopamine drives the ups and downs that can leave us vulnerable to overconsumption of all sorts. After a dopamine high, the dopamine crash can drop just as low as its previous heights—to even below our normal baseline level. The high and low points in this cycle leave us most vulnerable to the pleasures of food and other vices. Now that you know this, you can plan for it and intervene ahead of time. After all, that big to-do you're dreaming about is just another meal.

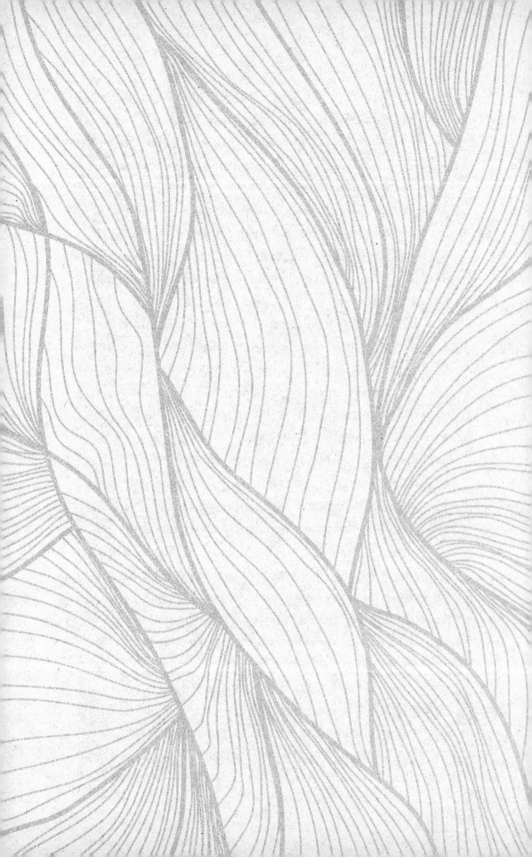

6.

~~~~~~~~

Carbohydrates and Dietary Fats: Demystifying the Darlings of Nutritional Science

I t's no wonder that carbs have such a bad rap in today's health culture. Mouthwatering starches and sugars can make everything from Grandma's cookies to your favorite breakfast scones addictive. They trigger cravings and are so, so easy to overconsume.

Mainstream thinking about how carbs and fat feed into obesity typically centers on two different models: "calories in, calories out" and the insulin-carbohydrate model, which proposes that a high-carbohydrate diet—including large amounts of refined starchy foods and sugar—causes release of too much insulin, which increases the storage of fat, which results in increased hunger, slowed metabolic rate, or both.[1] As always, the truth is likely somewhere in the middle. Now, let's unpack the science behind making the best carb and fat choices for your body.

CARBOHYDRATES

Most Americans get more than 50 percent of their calories from carbohydrates. And our collective overeating of starchy, sugary refined carbs has had devastating effects on our metabolism—resulting in rampant obesity, insulin resistance, and type 2 diabetes.[2]

The notion that packaged, processed foods can lead to nutritional imbalance probably comes as no surprise, but keep in mind that **whole grains, fruits, and vegetables count as carbs too**. Even whole grain-based carbs that have a low carb-to-fiber ratio can be a liability to your body composition. The more you eat, the easier it is to stress the insulin response, which amplifies the effects of overeating. I am not suggesting you should consume zero carbs; instead, I recommend strategic integration of carbohydrates into a balanced diet.

Carbohydrates come in two types: **fibrous** and **starchy/sugary**. Sugar is a small molecule, while both starches and fibers are made of long chains of simple sugar molecules. Because human digestive enzymes are unable to effectively break down fiber in plant foods, their consumption doesn't result in a blood-sugar response. Starches, on the other hand, are rapidly digested into sugar units and, practically speaking, have about the same effect as simple sugars on blood sugar. Mitigating blood-sugar spikes is one reason my patients learn to combine protein and/or fat with their carbs rather than eating carbs solo. While carbohydrate-containing foods, such as nonstarchy fibrous vegetables, are important for supporting the microbiome, the body does not require plant foods enriched in sugars and starches to meet its glucose requirements.

YOUR BODY CAN MAKE THE GLUCOSE IT NEEDS

Our bodies do have an absolute need for glucose, which provides an essential fuel for the brain, neurons, red blood cells, kidneys, and pancreas. This obligatory glucose totals approximately 80 to 100 grams of carbohydrates per day. Based on this need, the National Academy of Sciences established an RDA for carbohydrates of 130 grams per day. But this recommendation fails to account for the fact that glucose is not actually an essential *dietary* nutrient. **That's because *your body can make it*.**

Some AAs from protein are converted to glucose in the liver through a process called gluconeogenesis. For every 100 grams of protein consumed, roughly 60 grams of glucose are produced in the body.[3] By properly dosing your protein, your body can become efficient at generating its own glucose rather than constantly relying on dietary carbs. When you increase your dietary protein, you increase glucose production in a proportionate manner. And the benefits don't stop there! This approach also lowers triglycerides and increases HDL cholesterol. **Simply put, prioritizing dietary proteins while restricting carbohydrates can reverse metabolic syndrome.**

Although it's true that we don't need to consume carbohydrates to provide glucose as part of a healthy diet, we *do* need fiber. Fruits and vegetables are important sources of dietary fiber and micronutrients. **Soluble fiber**—the type found in citrus, apples, and oatmeal—isn't just good for your digestive system, but can also potentially decrease your total serum cholesterol.

Based on relevant research, the Lyon RDA for carbs calls for eating about 14 grams of fiber for every 1,000 calories you consume.[2] Rounding up a bit to make the math a little easier, a 200-pound man should aim for 30 grams of fiber daily, while a 140-pound woman should shoot for 25 grams. Now, how do you choose those grams wisely? Let's talk through the key ratios for determining the carb content of your diet.

QUALITY CARBS

To meet your goals without overconsuming calories, I recommend higher-fiber foods such as vegetables, berries, beans, and lentils. One advantage is that fiber slows digestion, keeping you full longer. In addition, high-fiber foods tend to also be whole foods found in nature, which are always my favorites. With my plan, two practical relationships drive dietary decision-making: the **ratio of carbs to protein** and the **ratio of carbs to fiber**.

The carb-to-protein ratio defines how many grams of carbohydrates you can have at a meal and still maintain metabolic balance. To promote weight loss, your overall dietary **carb-to-protein ratio** should be less than 1.0, far lower than the average American diet, which has a ratio of almost 5.0. (We'll discuss exactly how to apportion your macronutrients in chapter 7.) I also recommend that you never eat carbs alone; instead, combine them with either fat or preferably protein, ideally at least 10 grams. I always recommend that you "preload" with protein or fats before eating carbohydrates.

That pairing, along with fiber content, will determine carbohydrates' impact on your blood-sugar levels and insulin response. The carb-to-fiber ratio helps you gauge the quality of individual carbohydrate foods so you can favor ones that provide healthy fiber and avoid those that can contribute to weight gain. **Foods with a carb-to-fiber ratio of less than six have a low glycemic load and high levels of fiber.** (A ratio of 8:1 offers a bit more flexibility for those who tolerate carbs such as whole grains and starchier vegetables for a little more nutrient diversity.) These include most vegetables and berries.

Here are some examples of high-fiber carbs that I recommend based on these ratios:

- 1 cup of broccoli contains about 7.8 grams of carbs and 4.6 grams of fiber. Doing the math (7.8/4.6 = 1.7) shows a carb-to-fiber ratio for broccoli of 1.7.

- For green beans, the ratio is 2.5.
- Raspberries, 1.7.
- Strawberries, 3.1.
- Blueberries, 5.1.
- Most beans, 3.0.

Foods with carb-to-fiber ratios of about six or lower all constitute excellent plant-based food choices that can encourage fat loss while maintaining nutrient balance.

Foods to avoid or eat in moderation include potatoes, rice, pasta, and breads, which have carb-to-fiber ratios of 10 to 30, and fruits such as bananas and watermelon with carb-to-fiber ratios greater than 10. However, to a certain extent, you can have your cake and eat it too by leveraging resistant starch. Resistant starch, as the name implies, is resistant to digestion by our human enzymes, which means it impacts blood-sugar levels only minimally (an added bonus: it's great for the microbiome). As it turns out, you can reduce the glycemic loads of foods like white rice and potatoes by creating resistant starches.

To make resistant starch rice, cook white rice with a fat source like olive oil and then, after it's done cooking, cool the rice in the fridge. Together, the addition of fat and the cooling process catalyze the formation of resistant starch from the once simple starches present in this food.[4] The same can be done for potatoes, except the fat is added after cooking, followed by cooling.[5] Additionally, while ripe yellow bananas are high in sugar, green and semi-green bananas are enriched in resistant starch, making them better options from a blood-sugar perspective. And finally, cooked and cooled beans and chickpeas are another great source of both resistant starch and fiber, making them great selections from both blood-sugar and weight-management standpoints.

By understanding important properties of foods such as carb-to-protein ratio, carb-to-fiber ratio, and resistant-starch content, you can equip yourself with the information needed to create a customized fat-loss diet. (Stay tuned for more on exactly how to do this.)

Produce (per 100 g, raw unless specified)	Carbs (g)	Fiber (g)	Carb:Fiber
spinach	4.0	2.0	2.0
arugula	4.0	1.5	2.7
Swiss chard	4.0	2.0	2.0
collard greens	5.0	4.0	1.3
avocado	8.5	7.0	1.2
carrots	10.0	3.0	3.3
parsnips	18.0	5.0	3.6
beets	10.0	3.0	3.3
asparagus	4.0	2.0	2.0
eggplant, cooked	6.0	3.0	2.0
broccoli	7.0	3.0	2.3
cauliflower	5.0	3.0	1.7
Brussels sprouts	9.0	4.0	2.3
cabbage	6.0	2.5	2.4
sauerkraut	4.0	3.0	1.3
kimchi	2.5	1.5	1.7
white mushrooms	3.0	1.0	3.0
oyster mushrooms	6.0	2.0	3.0
zucchini	3.0	1.0	3.0
spaghetti squash	7.0	1.5	4.6
green beans	7.0	3.5	2.0
romaine lettuce	3.0	2.0	1.5
celery	3.0	1.5	2.0
tomatoes	4.0	1.0	4.0

Produce (per 100 g, raw unless specified)	Carbs (g)	Fiber (g)	Carb:Fiber
radishes	3.0	1.5	2.0
artichoke	11.0	5.0	2.2
green bell pepper	5.0	1.5	3.3
banana pepper	5.0	3.5	1.4
lentils (cooked)	20.0	8.0	2.5
chickpeas (cooked)	27.0	8.0	3.4
black beans (cooked)	24.0	9.0	2.7
edamame (cooked)	10.0	5.0	2.0
raspberries	12.0	7.0	1.7
blackberries	10.0	5.0	2.0
strawberries	8.0	2.0	4.0
wild blueberries	12.0	2.5	4.8
kiwi	15.0	3.0	5.0

CARBOHYDRATE TOLERANCE

A muscle-centric approach to health and longevity requires a protein-centered diet and **careful calculation of your meal tolerance for carbohydrates**. Recognizing your relationship with these foods will help you understand your personal flexibility. Some of my patients are so carb-addicted that they slip right into binge eating when they start with eating just a little. Becoming carbohydrate abstainers helps them disrupt the unhealthy pattern. How about you?

It helps to gauge carbohydrates based on a per-meal threshold. Proper dosing ranges between 20 and 40 grams (50 grams at the very high range without added exercise, but I don't typically go that high), depending on how you like to eat and the total carbs you consume in a day. The key is to ensure that your body uses all that you take in. Being able to get rid of the carbs we eat is called postprandial glucose clearance. This critical factor establishes our carbohydrate meal tolerance. To avoid post-meal elevations in blood glucose, or hyper-glycemia, a carbohydrate meal must be efficiently cleared within two hours. Glucose elevation beyond this time frame is the definition of diabetes. Remember, while we do need glucose, it has toxic effects if levels remain elevated for extended periods of time.

Once our muscles' glycogen stores are filled, it's time to empty them. Metabolic dysfunction and mitochondrial dysfunction within the skeletal muscle lead to decreased flux through glycogen and fat pools. Ultimately, type 2 diabetes results as a symptom of this decrease.

Skeletal muscle, as a primary site of insulin resistance, plays a huge role in blood-sugar regulation. In fact, problematic insulin resistance can begin in muscle tissue a decade before overt health problems appear. As we've seen in the previous pages, unhealthy muscle is a root cause of blood-glucose management problems, which set up a series of conditions that distort blood triglycerides and other markers.[6] My recommendation to consume 40 grams or less of net carbs per meal is informed by our understanding of the glucose-disposal rate given our goal to limit the insulin spike. Note that the *net carb* content of a given food is equal to the total carbs minus the number of grams of fiber.

Far too often, people remain sedentary immediately after meals. This limits glucose disposal into skeletal muscle to a baseline rate of approximately 3 grams of glucose per hour. After we account for glucose use by the brain, body, and liver, the two-hour post-meal disposal capacity equals approximately 50 grams. So this is where we start in healthy individuals.

As I mentioned earlier, the current RDA for carbohydrates is 130 grams per day, which provides for basic glucose fuel needs as well as allowing for five servings of vegetables, two to three servings of fruit, and three servings of whole grains.[7] Adults in the US typically consume nearly three times the RDA, or 300 grams per day. Still, fewer than 25 percent eat three servings of vegetables and two of fruit. You can see how this combination of high quantity and low quality sets up disastrous consequences.

One problem is a lack of clear guidance. It's obvious that excess carbohydrate intake is problematic and that dietary management of issues such as type 2 diabetes requires controlling meal carb intake as well as overall calorie management. Still, the American Diabetes Association asserts that "there is not a single ideal percentage of calories from carbohydrates, protein, and fats for all people with diabetes." General dietary guidelines recommend a nearly 4:1 ratio of carbohydrates to protein.[8] Meanwhile, the National Academy of Sciences defines the RDAs for carbohydrates and protein as 130 grams per day and around 65 grams per day, respectively, or a ratio of 2:1 carbohydrates to protein. At the same time, many clinical studies for controlling hyperglycemia of type 2 diabetes use a ratio of around 1:1.[9] Given this huge variability, no wonder people are confused!

The truth that no one is mentioning is this: **Success with any of these ranges depends on muscle health.** My goal is to streamline this information so that you can watch in real time as your body composition, hunger, and blood markers all improve by creating a meal threshold of 30 to 50 grams of high-quality carbs. You can do this!

At first, I suggest that you start by eating 90 grams of carbohydrates from whole-food sources daily, split over three meals. Then, as you become healthier, you can gradually increase this amount until you reach your personal carbohydrate threshold. Understand that we must start low and go slow. Healthy muscle can better manage carbs. By now, I hope you understand that you need to choose your carbs based on both quality and quantity and can see why you must earn through exercise any extra carbs in your carbohydrate budget.

SOFIA'S STORY

My patient Sofia originally came to me somewhat reluctantly, on assignment from a well-known food blog. A strong-willed and opinionated powerhouse, Sofia arrived skeptical and a bit defiant. Her editors had put her up to the task of regaining her health. Despite believing she was satisfied with her wellness level, she took on the challenge. When I asked about her reluctance, she acknowledged discomfort about being exposed publicly and having to face her daily habits and choices. Sofia's assignment wound up totally transforming her health and her life.

For Sofia, food was both a reward and a stress-relief strategy. She carried around about twenty pounds of extra fat, considered herself "big-boned," and had no regular exercise routine. That first day, she sauntered into my office, announcing, "OK, I have agreed to this, but let's be clear, I am perfectly happy with my weight, I am not giving up sugar and carbs, and I hate weight training."

Well, we are off to a good start, I thought to myself. In truth, I welcome resistance. It tells me exactly the area we need to lean into to push through.

"I don't want to be one of those people who are obsessed with their weight or how they look," Sofia continued.

I hear this a lot. My approach is to look for the conversation beneath the conversation. What she was really saying was (1) that focusing on herself made her uncomfortable, and (2) that she feared she could never reach the physical goals she really wished she could achieve. The buried inner monologue had been at work for years, and a lack of self-worth had restricted her willingness to try. Good thing for both of us, I was totally up for the challenge. I knew I'd have to operate strategically.

Despite her stated comfort with her current weight, Sofia's bloodwork told a different story. She had elevated inflammatory markers, low levels of key nutrients, and elevated cholesterol, insulin, and blood sugar—all at the tender age of thirty-five.

I knew the best approach would be to focus on mental framework by slowly showing her that she *could* make changes and become a better, healthier version of herself. Her mind would be sharp, her energy would be up, and her body would thank her. Over the year and a half that we worked together, she came in to see me monthly for a check-in and progress report. As she pushed through each level of mental resistance, which included all those old stories she'd repeated to herself, she became stronger and fitter. A new sense of confidence and leaning into physical challenge inspired her rather than pushing her away.

She took her success with physical challenges into the mental realm. She started placing candy on her desk to practice her resistance muscle. At one point in time, she'd believed that she *had* to eat what she saw. She was deeply tied to these old thoughts but found that when she put into place a new response, she no longer felt like a hostage.

This sense of agency transferred to all the "temptations" she faced. She became the boss of her own life. Every day, she chose one uncomfortable hurdle. Sometimes she'd test her ability to avoid checking her phone for a set number of hours. She'd walk rather than taking the subway. She skipped her midafternoon coffee. None of these trials was extreme, but they helped her practice not always choosing the "easy" thing. These subtle changes made a big impact in her life. Sofia went from acting on every desire to consciously choosing her actions and her restraints. She went from saying "I could never give up carbs" to "What's the big deal? How was I so attached to any one food?" As we balanced her blood sugar, she lost pounds of body fat and gained muscle. The most important thing she gained was her trust in herself.

A healthy approach to making responsible choices impacted every part of her life and psyche. She became the person she knew she could be and left nothing on the table. For fun, Sofia ran a marathon. She explored heavy-weight training and challenged herself with activities she had never tried before.

I am in the business of changing lives, and the modality I use is medicine. I seek freedom for my patients, and freedom is what they get. You can seize this same freedom in your own life. Learn how to do it your way on the pages to come!

THE SKINNY ON FAT

Fear of fats is the eight-hundred-pound gorilla behind the US Dietary Guidelines. No matter how the science changes, federal policymakers still seem to act as if fats are the root of all evil. Since the early 1970s, health-care professionals have obsessed over the idea that fats and cholesterol contribute to virtually all health problems, including heart disease, obesity, diabetes, and cancer. While the fat theory might *seem* logical, the evidence is based on educated guesses, assumptions, and personal beliefs. After nearly fifty years of research, the case against dietary fat has yet to be proven—in fact, the evidence gets weaker with each passing day.

The two theories behind the belief that fat is bad for health are that (1) cholesterol causes heart disease because artery-clogging plaque contains cholesterol, and (2) fat makes you fat because, well . . . it just seems logical, doesn't it?

Both theories have been proven wrong,[10] but big food and pharmaceutical companies make lots of money selling highly processed plant oils chemically turned into margarines, shortenings, and hydrogenated oils, along with prescription drugs such as statins. If you didn't believe these fake theories about fat, then you wouldn't buy all those processed foods and the medicines, right?

When choosing between fats, keep in mind that all are not created equal. Dietary fats come in four types: monounsaturated, polyunsaturated, saturated, and trans fats, each with different impacts on health.

Unsaturated Fats

Predominantly found in plant foods, such as vegetable oils, nuts, and seeds, unsaturated fats are considered helpful for improving blood-cholesterol levels and easing inflammation, along with other benefits.

Sources of **monounsaturated fats** include:
- Olives
- Avocados
- Nuts, including almonds, hazelnuts, and pecans
- Seeds such as pumpkin and sesame

Sources of **polyunsaturated fats** include:
- Walnuts
- Flaxseeds
- Fish
- Fish roe
- Shellfish

Among the polyunsaturated fats are essential fatty acids, which may provide the biggest health benefits.[11] Data show that substituting polyunsaturated fats for saturated fats in patients with metabolic syndrome is associated with greater reductions in triglycerides than using monounsaturated fats, independent of weight loss. These findings raise the possibility that polyunsaturated fats could reduce cardiometabolic risk in these patients. Remember, when we choose our calories wisely, polyunsaturated fats are the ones to prioritize.

For muscle health, protein and carbohydrates are the primary nutrients of concern. But essential fatty acids such as omega-3s also play an important role. Omega-3 fatty acids are a group of essential polyunsaturated fats that need to come from dietary sources since the body can't make them. These have numerous health benefits (think of omega-3 as "vitamin F" for "fatty acids").[12] Supplementation with fish-oil-derived omega-3 has been shown to improve body composition, muscle strength, physical performance, and serum lipid profiles in older adults.[13] These results suggest increasing omega-3s could prove to be helpful in preventing sarcopenia.

While fishes offer the richest animal-based sources, plant sources of omega-3s include algal oil supplements, flaxseeds, pumpkin seeds, and walnuts. Omega-3 fatty acids come in three forms: plant-derived alpha-linolenic acid (ALA), animal-derived eicosapentaenoic acid (EPA), and docosahexaenoic acid (DHA). Over the past three centuries, American food-supply changes have led to decreases in omega-3 consumption, along with increases in total fat and omega-6 fatty acid intake. The result: a huge shift in the omega-6/omega-3 ratio, from 1:1 in the agricultural period to greater than 20:1 today, which can have significant inflammatory effects.[14] Modern agriculture's focus on food quantity over quality has led to animal-feed changes, decreasing the omega-3 fatty acid content in commonly available foods such as meats, eggs, and even fish, making it more challenging for us to consume sufficient levels.

How livestock are raised has an impact on the composition of their fat tissue. Animals fed grain-based and feedlot diets are enriched with omega-6 fatty acids (which may be needed to help demands of growth). This increase in omega-6 can distort the balance of the omega-3/omega-6 ratio, even though livestock are not our primary dietary source of omega-6 fatty acids. While no single food is the problem, I do believe that excess amounts of omega-6 compared with omega-3 are problematic. To correct this imbalance, focus on eating foods rich in omega-3. If wild-caught or grass-fed, grass-finished land-animal products seem beyond your budget, try choosing salmon from Scotland or small, wild-caught fish such as sardines or mackerel. Given all the unknowns, I also recommend adding a fish, algal, or krill oil to your daily regimen. Or consume conventional beef and add in an omega-3 supplement.

Saturated Fat

Let's shift gears to the biggest fat attention-grabber of the past several decades: saturated fat. Over millions of years, the only fat that humans or other mammals evolved to make is saturated fat, because it is highly stable and resistant to oxidative damage. If saturated fat were as toxic as current common wisdom implies, we would all be dead. **Dietary saturated fats become a risk only if you're overconsuming calories and carbohydrates.**

While high saturated-fat concentrations are primarily found in animal-based foods (such as butter, cheese, and red meat), they are also present in certain plant-based foods (specifically coconut and tropical oils made from coconut, palm, and palm kernels). These days, modern, economically driven agricultural practices, such as grain-feeding instead of grass-feeding livestock, lead to animal products that contain more saturated fat. Still, the predominant fat in both grass- and grain-fed cattle is monounsaturated, followed by saturated fat, one-third of which is a neutral fat called stearin that doesn't raise cholesterol. Remember, saturated fat itself does not pose a problem. Instead, its calorie density can lead to intake of too many calories if overconsumed. For this reason, I recommend eating the leanest cuts available.

While I'm not one to demonize fat the way many did in the 1980s, I'm also not on the high-fat bandwagon. Fat density matters, and choosing low-fat options helps keep calories in check. After all, we don't consume macronutrients individually, filling our plates with a couple of squares of saturated fat plus a pile of protein and a small side of carbs. That's not how food works. Instead, we must make informed choices about the micro- and macronutrient combinations that each food provides to strike a healthy balance at each meal and throughout a day.

Because eating extra saturated fat provides no benefits and can instead lead to increased caloric intake, it's important to take care with your consumption. We know that saturated fat can raise LDL cholesterol in some people. I recommend replacing saturated with unsaturated fats, especially polyunsaturated, whenever possible. Review of evidence by the American Heart Association concluded that this replacement lowers the incidence of cardiovascular disease.[15]

To truly understand cholesterol, it's critical to recognize that it is essential for life and fundamental to the structure of every cell in your body—from your brain to your skin. To stay alive, we need 1,000 milligrams daily of cholesterol, which is so essential that our bodies evolved to make it. Most people make about 800 milligrams a day in the liver and consume about 200 milligrams a day from dietary sources. If you have a cholesterol problem, it's a problem with either the rate at which the liver makes cholesterol or the rate at which it removes cholesterol from the blood. The research is absolutely clear: blood cholesterol is not related to dietary cholesterol.

Trans Fat

Before we move on, let's dispense with trans fats, most of which get manufactured in an industrial process that uses hydrogen to solidify vegetable oils. You'll find trans fats in spreads (such as margarine), baked goods (including store-bought pastries, muffins, and cookies), and fried foods (french fries, chicken nuggets, doughnuts, and others). Steer clear of trans fats, which increase your risks for heart disease, stroke, and type 2 diabetes.[16]

■

Many popular diets recommend restricting dietary fat overall and avoiding saturated fats, mostly because fats have a higher calorie content (9 calories per gram). But fats also have a higher satiety value, meaning they tend to leave you feeling full, unlike carbohydrates, which can make you hungry, convincing you there's always room for dessert even when you're stuffed. Remember, weight management and body fat are determined by the number of calories you eat. That's why it's so important to master balancing your macronutrients for optimal health. Instead of obsessing over saturated fats, focus on polyunsaturated fats to get in those essential omega-3s.

Fat is a very efficient fuel for skeletal muscle, and individual fatty acids are essential for every cell membrane—especially the unique protective layer around nerve structures in our brains. This makes fatty acids an essential requirement, but the minimum amount we need is very low, only about 3 grams of essential fatty acids per day. Diet-wise, **that translates to eating between 25 and 35 percent of our daily** calories from fat to get the minimum 3 grams of essential fatty acids. Of course, you can drop this a bit lower to 20 percent or increase up to 40 percent.

Consuming no less than 30 grams of fat per day is ideal for most people. Maintaining this midrange level helps with satiety, which, as anyone who's been "on a diet" can tell you, is key to lasting success.

MINDSET RESET

RECLAIM YOUR RIGHT TO HEALTH

Reclaiming your right to good health requires breaking down any barriers standing in your way. Be forewarned that this process will unearth all sorts of internal protests. Not to worry. All that naysaying chatter is just your inner monologue attempting to negotiate a way out of the discomfort that comes with growth and change. Anticipating challenges, developing practical strategies, and harnessing your own inner strength will help you deliver, almost effortlessly, on your new wellness habits until those habits become your identity.

This is the approach I took with my patient Ava. When it came to work, Ava was always extremely disciplined. A successful real estate agent with her own firm, she was a pro at creating better outcomes for others yet struggled to do the same for herself. Despite "eating healthy and exercising," Ava, forty-seven, had struggled with obesity since childhood. Worried about a future full of medical issues, she came to me in tears, close to giving up any hope of balancing her body composition and metabolism. Once we dove deep into imagining what it might take for her to create a better future for herself, it became clear that she needed to apply the skills and qualities she'd honed through her career toward improving her own health.

Ava's situation is one I see often: a highly successful person, dialed into their work, who spends all their effort and energy on anything and everything except their health. (I'm sure you know people like this—or maybe this is YOU?) Step one in these cases is to explore the beliefs that stand in the way of self-care. Exploring Ava's existing mental framework helped us identify the biggest barrier thwarting her progress: she didn't feel worthy of good health and extraordinary fitness. My job was to instill in her the confidence to advocate for her own health the way she so successfully advocated for clients. I helped her see that this person, committed to self-care, had been a part of her all along. We nurtured her best self, then worked to ensure the results that would keep her motivated and on track over the long term.

Gay Hendricks calls this an "upper limit problem." In his book *The Big Leap*, he explains that we all have a threshold for feeling good, how much health improvement (fat loss, metabolic correction, etc.) we feel worthy of attaining.[17] A restricted sense of self will convince you to look outward to place blame. This can leave you hating who you are, with no idea how you wound up scrolling through social media comparing yourself with others and coming away feeling less-than. If you've ever felt defeated and wondered why you even try, it's time to swap out that old, clouded lens for a clear one.

For Ava, working past this upper limit of self-worth took daily practice and visualization. Eventually, she learned how to care for herself as much as she did for others. Once she internalized a sense of worthiness, she was able to commit to the changes that turned her life around.

To prioritize her workouts, we placed boundaries on her work in the evening. To help her invest more energy and attention into her training, we banned her from using her phone in the gym. Ava also needed to learn to eat with intentionality instead of mindlessness. We slowed everything down. To replace the takeout she ordered regularly, we planned her meals, and she cooked in bulk to make it super easy to maintain her food plan. She stopped starving herself and yo-yo dieting. Instead, she ate whole foods and tracked her calories. She wrote her training and meals into her calendar and gave them the same attention she granted to clients. The focus of our work was not weight loss but mindful execution of her plan to help keep her on track mentally and physically. We focused on building positive momentum with weekly check-ins. With these support structures in place, Ava stayed accountable and committed, slimmed down, built muscle, and slept better. The weight she lost was not just excess fat but also the burden of shame and low self-esteem.

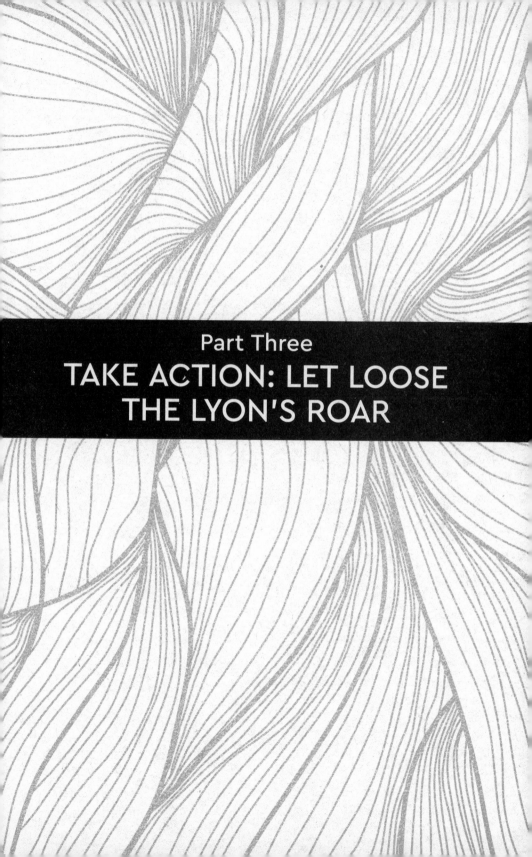

Part Three
TAKE ACTION: LET LOOSE THE LYON'S ROAR

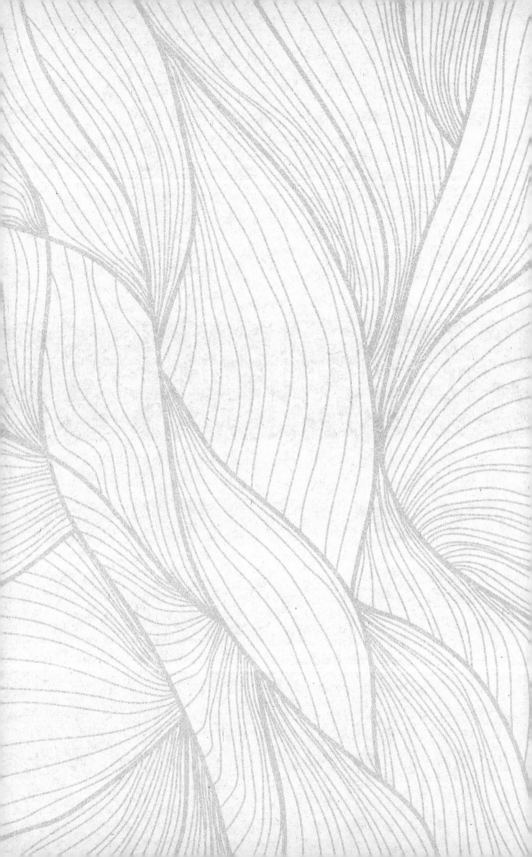

7.

〜〜〜〜〜

The Lyon Protocol Meal Plans

Now it's time to implement all that you've learned. Here's where I help you design a balanced, protein-forward diet that I am sure will help you control your hunger, metabolism, and longevity. I have treated thousands of patients, offering the same recommendations that I'm about to give you. The amazing part about switching to an eating plan that targets protein for muscle health is seeing immediate results. Consistently optimizing your protein intake will reduce cravings, balance blood sugar, improve muscle tone, supercharge energy, and improve mental clarity. You'll start to enjoy these benefits right away.

Many people starting a new protocol have two main concerns: Will I feel hungry? Will this be sustainable? I assure you that you'll not feel as hungry as you probably have with other diets, and yes, these protocols are not only manageable but easily enjoyed over the course of a lifetime. **The Lyon Protocol is not a diet but an educated lifestyle.** Our focus is on intelligent muscle health—a way of refining your intake and output to align with your ultimate health mission, whether it is graceful aging, a great body, or maintaining mental and physical strength over the decades.

Living a protein-forward lifestyle supports healthy weight loss by working synergistically with exercise to protect skeletal muscle while losing fat. Now is the time for us to dig into the dietary details of meal planning.

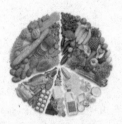

HOW TO CALCULATE YOUR DAILY
MACRONUTRIENT TARGETS

High-quality protein is the basis for any nutrition plan. Your goal is to take in at least 1 gram of protein per pound of ideal body weight, keeping in mind that every protein gram contains 4 calories. Whether you're trying to bulk up or lose fat, 30 to 50 grams of protein per meal will help maintain your skeletal muscle mass. This recommendation is based on consuming the right amount of essential amino acids, such as leucine, to optimize muscle-protein synthesis. All high-quality (i.e., animal-based) protein is interchangeable. Every ounce of food from land mammals contains 7 grams of protein, while fish contains 5 grams of protein per ounce. Gauging protein in terms of a percentage of diet is outdated thinking. Protein should remain stable or increase when calories are decreased, as it is essential to protect muscle and other tissues.

Next, let's determine your carbohydrates. Given all the strong opinions and crazy fad diets governing carbs, many people find them the most confusing macro. You've likely encountered dietary guidelines that recommend carbohydrate intakes of 45 to 65 percent of your daily calories. This might be appropriate if you're an elite athlete or a highly active construction worker, but for most adults, consuming this many carbohydrates will provide far too many calories. So let's take an approach more suited to modern American lifestyles. If you're metabolically healthy, aim for a carb-to-protein ratio of 1:1, and keep your carb grams around 30 to 50 grams per meal to minimize the insulin response. If your training program includes extended bouts of exercise (where your heart rate reaches above at least 120 beats per minute), you can incorporate additional carbohydrates—perhaps an additional 60 grams per hour of moderate to intense exercise. If you are less active, you should stick within the daily 90 to 130 grams range. For anyone overweight or who has abnormal blood markers showing carb intolerance, I recommend limiting starches and grains to no more than 30 grams per day to start. Then use the rest of your carb budget for leafy greens, red and orange vegetables, or high-fiber fruits like berries.

Finally, let's define our goal for fat. Fat makes up every cell membrane, including the unique protective layer around nerve structures in our brains. It also provides important fuel for muscle. Practically speaking, when it comes to apportioning macros, fats and carbohydrates are interchangeable. Start by identifying your protein goal, see how many

calories that equates to, and then move on to set your carbohydrate total based on your activity level. Whatever remaining
calories you have left can be dedicated toward healthy fats. As
you read in chapter 6, too much fat can wind up driving up
calories (and possibly LDL cholesterol) and/or displacing protein in your diet. Keep fat calories within your overall calorie
budget. As a guideline, the remaining daily fat allowance typically falls between 0.7 and 2.2 grams per kilogram of body
weight. Note that fat contains 9 calories per gram and can be
interchangeable with carbohydrates based on your personal
preferences and caloric intake. Making healthy food choices
should keep you on track with your fat intake.

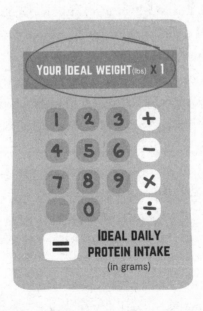

MACRONUTRIENT RECOMMENDATIONS

➡ 1g of protein per every pound of ideal body weight

➡ 1:1 carb-to-protein ratio (for metabolically healthy individuals)

➡ 0.7–2.2 grams/kg daily fat intake

Now it's time to put these building blocks to work. Here are some of my recommendations for incorporating good-quality carbohydrates, proteins, and fats into your diet:

- Always select high-quality food sources. Avoid ultra-processed foods in bags or boxes. Buy fresh vegetables, fruits, meats, dairy, and eggs.
- Prioritize vegetable-based carb sources. You can add in some starches around workouts or if they fit your macros.
- Weigh your food. Do you have to do this forever? No, but you are training yourself to figure out exactly what you're eating. Learn what portion size is appropriate for you. The more practice you get visualizing your eating, the quicker you can ditch the scale—if you remember what your plates typically look like.

Commit yourself to taking these important steps. Sure, you might deviate for a special occasion, but don't let periodic exceptions derail your overall consistency. Let this guide serve as a template for life.

Trying to lose weight without tracking your food is like setting out on a voyage without a compass.

STRATEGIES FOR MEAL PLAN SUCCESS

Before jumping into your chosen meal protocol, here are a few imperatives that will help ensure success:

❶ Find a consistent eating schedule. Food impacts your body's circadian cycles, and this allows your body to create a schedule. Do not get distracted by food. Stick to your plan.

❷ Avoid chaotic, haphazard eating. Plan your meals ahead of time. Pack and store what you need to make sure you're ready to start the week.

❸ If you really want to see change, limit dining out. The less food eaten away from home, the better. If you do go to a restaurant, plan your choices ahead of time by looking at menus beforehand.

❹ Manage your expectations. The magic of any goal worth achieving comes through sustained effort and hard work.

❺ Expect your mind's chatter to try to talk you out of your goals. Dominate the mental monologue.

❻ Develop the discipline to push yourself.

❼ Know your weaknesses, and plan for them. Following predesigned game plans will lead you to victory.

With this approach, you will immediately begin managing hunger and protecting your bones, organs, and muscles. **You will see and feel changes right away, with improvements noticeable after just one meal!** Still, your short-term choices from meal to meal will determine the long game. To help you choose your path based on your objectives, I will outline three improvement tracks and an overview of what each entails. These plans focus on optimizing **longevity, body composition,** and **muscle mass,** respectively. Rotating through each of these three plans will grant you access to a legacy of wellness.

Step one is to get honest with yourself about how much you're eating now. Let's start by crunching the numbers to do some metabolic math.

METABOLIC MATH
Keep it simple. Keep it clean. Keep it disciplined.

How many calories do you need in a day? To figure out how much you should eat in a day, we need to assess your starting place. Start by determining the total calories you'd need to simply maintain your status quo, keeping your current weight and body composition. If your weight is currently relatively stable, that means you're eating at a "caloric maintenance" level. Caloric maintenance refers to the number of calories you would need to consume to maintain your current body weight. Weighing and tracking your food are imperative to determining an accurate number.

 Track your food for two to four typical weeks. I recommend plugging these numbers into an app like Cronometer that focuses on tallying both macro- and micronutrients. Assuming your weight is stable, the data you gather after two to four typical weeks will reveal your maintenance calories.

> Based on tracking two to four typical weeks,
> my maintenance calories total =_____.

Your maintenance calories show your status quo. Changing your body composition will require you to reallocate/add/subtract calories from your diet. Your recommended caloric intake depends on factors such as sex, age, and activity level. Most women need 1,600 to 2,400 daily calories to maintain their weight. Men typically need 2,000 to 3,000 calories. Eating fewer calories within your proper macro allocations will lead to fat loss without sacrificing muscle. Eating more calories that prioritize protein will support muscle gain.

If you are an analytic type, you might like this alternative calculation.

A "quick and dirty" method of determining your recommended daily caloric intake, based solely on total body weight and desired outcome, can be calculated using one of these formulas:

- Fat loss = 12 to 13 calories per pound of ideal body weight
- Maintenance = 15 to 16 calories per pound of current body weight
- Weight gain = 18 to 19 calories per pound of current body weight

Example: *Because I weigh 115 pounds, my maintenance calories can be determined as follows: 115 lb × 15 kcal = 1,725 kcal per day.*

Alternatively, the Harris-Benedict Calculator (https://www .inchcalculator.com/harris-benedict-calculator) is a great option if you want a quick starting place and don't yet know how many calories you're currently eating. As you track your caloric consumption over time, you can start to learn and make visual adjustments based on portion sizes.

BASAL METABOLIC RATE

While we're on the topic of metabolic math, another important parameter to consider is basal metabolic rate (BMR), the total calories your body needs to keep up with basic life-sustaining functions. **BMR is not a goal to target but the bare minimum amount of energy that your body needs to fuel itself.** Once you know your BMR, you could estimate the total calories you should consume daily to meet your body-composition goals over time using an alternative metric called total daily energy expenditure (TDEE). **TDEE is the total number of calories that your body expends in a twenty-four-hour period,** including all physical activity along with your BMR.

Remember, there is NO one correct way to calculate how many daily calories you should consume. It's important to keep in mind that all the tools I've presented above can provide only estimates. Determining caloric intake is a moving target, and the trial and error of optimizing your consumption is an integral part of the process. Your priority now is to choose one of these options and take action.

Based on my goals to *lose/gain* (circle one) weight,
my recommended calories total =_____.

Now that you've ascertained your caloric needs, it's time to reach your goal. At the outset, it might seem difficult to determine what your ideal weight and muscle-mass numbers should be. Can you remember a time in your life when you looked and felt your best? Start there. That's a good place to set your sights. Next, it's time to formulate your macronutrient requirements. As always, we start with protein.

SAMPLE CALCULATION

SARA

140-pound perimenopausal woman

Goal weight: 125 pounds

Current body fat: 35%

Maintenance calories = 2,100 kcal, determined from four weeks of food tracking

To encourage weight loss, we create a calculated caloric deficit of 20%:

2,100 kcal × 0.20 = 420 kcal

2,100 kcal − 420 kcal = 1,680 kcal

Thus, Sara's recommended daily caloric intake for weight loss totals 1,680 kcal.

The next step is to calculate protein. Sara's goal weight is 125 pounds, which tells us her daily protein target totals 125 g. There are 4 kcal per gram of protein, which means she should consume 125 g × 4 kcal/g or 500 kcal of protein daily.

This protein should be distributed evenly across meals, so roughly 40 grams of protein three times per day, or three meals with 30 grams of protein plus snacks equating to an additional 30 grams of protein.

After accounting for protein calories, Sara has 1,180 calories remaining. She had been on a Standard American Diet (SAD) with a daily carbohydrate intake of easily 300 grams. So, to help her adjust to new eating patterns, we will allocate for her a 1:1 ratio of carbs to protein.

Factoring in 125 grams of carbs means that we have now accounted for an additional 500 kcal, as there are 4 kcal per gram of carbohydrate.

Because Sara's calories from protein and carbs total 1,000 kcal, she is now left with 680 kcal to ration toward fat. Fat contains 9 kcal per gram, so Sara can consume 680 kcal divided by 9 kcal/g or roughly 75 grams of fat.

Thus, Sara's final macro split is 125 grams protein, 125 grams carbs, and 75 grams fat.

Stay tuned to see how this macro split translates into actual food.

INSTRUCTIONS FOR BUILDING YOUR DIET AROUND PROTEIN

Keeping your protein consumption steady and on target is a nonnegotiable priority of the Lyon Protocol. Protein should be the first macronutrient you eat from your plate. Relative to protein, carbs and fat are completely negotiable. If you stick within your calorie budget, you can pick and choose between them based on your preferences.

Unlike with carbohydrates and dietary fats, calories from protein are nearly impossible to store as fat and almost always lead to improvement of body composition. A clear distinction between overeating carbs and overeating protein was drawn by Dr. Jose Antonio in a review published in the *International Journal of Exercise Science*.[1] "Overfeeding on carbohydrate and/or fat results in body composition alterations that are different than overfeeding on protein," Antonio observed, refuting the common belief that "3,500 kcal is equivalent to 0.45 kg (1 pound) of fat and that changing energy balance in accordance with this will produce predictable changes in body weight." Existing literature, he explained, does not support that conclusion.

Instead, **protein appears to have a protective effect against fat gain** during times of energy surplus (i.e., overeating), and this effect has an even bigger impact when combined with resistance training. Evidence suggests that **dietary protein may be the key macronutrient in terms of promoting positive changes in body composition**. Dietary protein's ability to fortify your muscular armor is why I recommend the simple formula, for nearly everyone, young and old, of consuming 1 gram of protein for each pound of your ideal body weight.

JUMP-START YOUR DAY WITH PROTEIN

There's some truth to the saying that breakfast is the most important meal of the day. A key element of the Lyon Protocol's ability to empower your body to protect lean tissues while supporting fat loss lies within the first meal after your overnight fast. Without sufficient signaling from leucine (the essential amino acid we discussed earlier), our muscles will interpret a meal as inadequate for supporting the nutrient demands of protein synthesis. Instead, the body will store the meal calories as fat while muscle breakdown continues until adequate protein is consumed. Eating enough protein at breakfast to promote protein synthesis will set you up for wins over the short and long term.

The work of Dr. Heather Leidy indicates that eating a protein-heavy first meal will change your eating patterns for the rest of the day. In her study, twenty overweight or obese adolescent females ages eighteen to twenty were broken up into three cohorts. Cohort 1 skipped breakfast, cohort 2 ate cereal (13 grams of protein), and cohort 3 consumed a high-protein (35 grams) breakfast consisting of eggs and lean beef. Leidy matched each breakfast for dietary fat, fiber, and sugar, and each contained 350 calories. The only differences between breakfasts were the macros in the protein and carbohydrate groups. The high-protein breakfast group received a 1:1 balance of protein to carbs, whereas the cereal-for-breakfast group received 13 grams of protein and 57 grams of carbs, for a protein-to-carb ratio of 1:4. Before dinner, a brain scan using functional magnetic resonance imaging tracked the neurological signals that control food motivation and reward-driven eating behavior. What they found was astonishing.

Members of the high-protein breakfast group felt more fullness or "satiety," and their brain activity suggested decreased food cravings. Compared with the groups eating a cereal breakfast or skipping it altogether, the high-protein breakfast group also snacked less on high-fat and high-sugar foods in the evening. Here's the takeaway: eating protein-rich foods for your first meal of the day will help quell cravings later, when high-fat or high-sugar snacks can be most tempting. Thus, **one easy strategy to prevent overeating and improve diet quality is prioritizing high-protein foods at breakfast.**

GUIDELINES FOR CARB CONTROL

Carbohydrate control is the next consideration on our list. To avoid the consequences of excess carbohydrates that can send blood-glucose levels soaring and drive inflammation and metabolic stress, be wary of carbohydrate intake at each meal, especially breakfast.

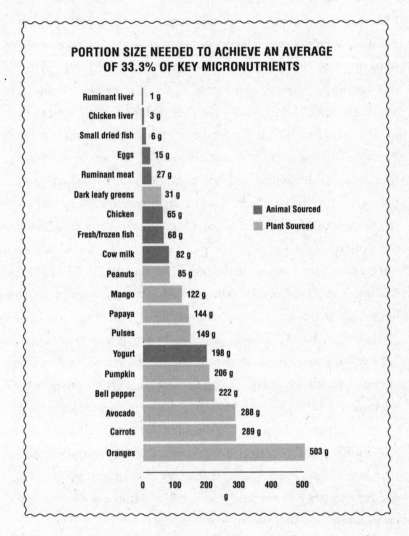

Portion size needed to achieve an average of 33.3 percent of requirements for iron, vitamin A, zinc, folate, vitamin B$_{12}$, and calcium, key micronutrients that are commonly lacking in the diets of low- and middle-income countries,[2] from complementary foods in Kenya (each micronutrient capped at 100 percent of daily requirements).

Carbohydrate control begins with making well-informed choices. Pick the carbs you like, prioritizing selections with carb-to-fiber ratios of less than six. (See the chart on page 144 that shows the ratios we utilized in Dr. Layman's lab, which I still use in my current clinical practice.) The other factors to consider are polyphenols and other phytonutrients that are known to boost health. These beneficial components are why I personally prefer carbs over fats. Factoring in carbs before fats provides me with a more fibrous and micronutrient-rich diet. So long as you are healthy, active, and hitting your protein needs, you can adjust your ratio of carbs to fats interchangeably. Just make sure to keep total carb quantities in check. To minimize insulin response, eat no more than 50 grams of carbs at any one time, and always pair them with protein and some fat.

Another benefit of carbohydrates is muscle hypertrophy. I choose foods not just for their fiber content but also for the robust amounts of other bioactive compounds in nutrient-dense plant foods that may help to regulate inflammation, muscle health, and many other processes in the body. I have included a table outlining plant foods with ideal carb-to-fiber ratios to help guide your choices.

FAT FACTS AND FIGURES

Humans have an essential need for certain fats, but figuring fat into your diet can be challenging because not all types affect the body equally. My primary goal is to afford you food flexibility while keeping your calories in check. Rarely do I focus on *adding* fat to a patient's diet. As I've mentioned, your first job is to set your protein goal before allocating your remaining calories to carbs and then fat. As a guideline, the fat calories remaining typically fall between 0.7 and 2.2 grams per kilogram of body weight per day.

WILD FOR THE WIN

Many edible wild plants contain a good balance of omega-6 and omega-3 fatty acids. Purslane, sometimes considered a weed, contains eight times more alpha-linolenic acid (ALA) than spinach, red-leaf lettuce, buttercrunch lettuce, or mustard greens. Moreover, bioactive food matrix values are much higher in wild plants such as wild blueberries than in their cultivated counterparts.[3]

Modern aquaculture's efforts to supply a larger population and keep costs low have changed fish's nutritional profile. Farmed fish contains significantly less omega-3 fatty acids than fish raised naturally in the ocean, rivers, and lakes.[4]

Meanwhile, the fatty-acid composition of egg yolks from free-range chickens has an omega-6/omega-3 ratio of 1.3, whereas a USDA egg has a ratio of 19.9.[5] By enriching chicken feed with fish meal or flaxseed, the ratio of omega-6 to omega-3 decreased to 6.6 and 1.6, respectively.

This is why it's important to eat a mix of pastured and wild animal proteins and bright local and seasonal fruits and vegetables.

OK, it's almost time to pick your meal plan protocol from three health-optimization improvement tracks. But first, a few words about hedonic eating.

Being able to discern eating for sport (hedonic eating) from actual hunger will determine your outcome 100 percent. The habits that surround nutrient intake are just as important as the nutrients you take in, so be mindful about what you put in your mouth and avoid using food as a tool for distraction. The long-term implications of hedonic eating are devastating, so it's key to become intimately familiar with

IS IT HEDONIC EATING
OR
ARE YOU REALLY HUNGRY?

HEDONIC	**PHYSICAL**
Bored/Distracting	Caloric Deficit
Habitual	Low Blood Sugar
Emotional/Stressed	Rumbling Stomach
Crave Specific Foods	Nonpleasurable Drive to Eat
Overeats	Stops Eating When Full

your cues of physical hunger. Eating in response to physical hunger is the beginning of a winning strategy.

AT LAST! It's time to incorporate everything you've learned so far to move forward and choose your nutritional plan.

PROTOCOL DESIGN

1. Pick your protocol.
2. Determine your baseline caloric needs.
3. Take the eating-style assessments and weakness assessments to build the global strength of your protocol.
4. Determine your daily total protein calories.
5. Determine your daily carbohydrate calories.
6. Determine your daily fat calories.
7. Build out your plan.

In this protocol, your goals will be determined by one of three choices: **optimize longevity**, **optimize body composition**, or **optimize muscle**. Once you've chosen your path, we can determine how many calories you need to reach your goal. With this starting point in place, you pick your protocol and build it out.

EATING-STYLE QUIZ

This (nonscientific) quiz is designed to help you get clarity about your own preferences, based on both your current reality and your goals for the future. Some of us are better at utilizing and burning fat, while others are better at utilizing carbs. Because you will gauge this while living your life (rather than sequestered in a metabolic ward), your findings will be somewhat subjective. This is where the art of the Lyon Protocol comes in.

How do you like to eat? How do those choices make you feel? How do they align with your health goals? If the answers to these questions are operating outside of your awareness, you can't make the intentional changes necessary for future wellness. Here's your chance to take ownership.

Determine your protein appetite.

Do you prefer eating more or less protein? _____

Which proteins are your favorites? _____

Determine your carbohydrate/fat tolerance.

Do you prefer to use your remaining calories for carbohydrates or fats? _____

Are you a carb lover, generally speaking? _____

What kinds of carbs do you prefer? _____

Does your body feel and look better when you eat more carbohydrates or more fats? _____

THE THREE HEALTH-OPTIMIZATION TRACKS

1. OPTIMIZE LONGEVITY

This plan is designed for people looking to live a longer, healthier life. Even adults who maintain a relatively steady body weight and generally seem healthy can have weak and insufficient muscle mass as well as excess body fat. Muscle deficiencies can show up as fatigue or low energy during regular daily routines, as well as abnormalities in clinical blood biomarkers such as lipids or glucose. By following a muscle-centric lifestyle—with targeted macronutrient intake and regular resistance training—many people can reverse these conditions, live long, and feel great while they're doing it.

The Optimizing Longevity Plan assumes that you are happy with your body composition yet confused about all the discussion in the longevity space. This track provides you with a plan for how to choose nutrient-dense foods in balanced ratios that will keep your muscles in good condition. It will also provide you with sustained energy. With no change in overall calories, this plan focuses on corrective macronutrients and nutrient density, choosing foods with a diversity of bioactive compounds. You will know exactly what you are eating and why. Knowledge is your health currency.

Optimize Longevity Plan Details:
- Two main meals plus one midday snack.
- Overall protein quantities can be increased to meet your overall protein goal once your body's needs have been clearly established.
- This plan can include a one-to-one ratio of carbs to protein if desired, but success depends on an individual's carbohydrate tolerance.

- REMINDER: I recommend consuming no less than 100 grams of protein daily for any adult, regardless of size.
- The core principle of the plan is reworking your current maintenance calories.

PROTEIN: 1.2 to 2.2 g/kg (0.7 to 1.0 g/lb)

CARBS: Determine your carbohydrate intake. Assuming you are metabolically healthy, your carb intake at baseline will range from 90 to 130 grams, or a carb-to-protein ratio of around 1:1. You can add 60 grams per day of carbs per hour of moderate- to high-intensity exercise. To minimize insulin response, keep from exceeding 40 to 50 grams of carbohydrates per meal on days that you're not exercising.

FAT: 0.7 to 2.2 g/kg (0.32 to 1.0 g/lb). The remainder of your calories can be dedicated to fats.

Ensure that your first meal of the day contains a minimum of 40 to 50 grams of protein, sufficient to trigger the leucine threshold. The overnight fast primes the body for a robust response to this first protein dose that will optimize muscle health. Keep carbohydrates at or below 30 grams in this first meal.

A small midday protein snack should contain at least 10 grams of protein with either carbs or fat, *if* these fall within your calorie budget. This snack is not designed to have a muscle effect but rather to keep hunger at bay. The snack can have a higher amount of protein, but that isn't necessary.

The second (last) meal of the day should contain roughly 50 grams of protein or more, depending on your protein goal, plus 50 grams or less of carbohydrates and fat as needed—unless you are participating in an intense exercise program. If you are exercising, you may increase your carbohydrates per meal for exercise recovery. Eating a protein-rich meal before the overnight fast will protect your muscle tissue.

As always, we start with the critical macronutrient: protein. Research has established a minimum amount of protein for muscle maintenance in the general population of 1.2 to 2.2 g/kg per day.[6] I recommend 2.2 g/kg if you're an athlete or looking to reduce your carbohydrate intake. This equals 0.54 to 1.0 g/lb. Keep in mind that if your diet is more plant-based, these numbers need to reach the higher end to meet your minimum amino-acid requirements. The maintenance number does not factor in whether stress to the body makes this less than optimal, but it will work. Again, I recommend no less than 100 grams of protein daily for any adult, regardless of size.

If you weigh 130 pounds and are happy with your weight and body composition, the minimum amount of protein you should consume totals 0.54 to 0.70 g/lb, which would put you at the lowest end: 70 to 91 grams of protein. However, if you understand the concepts laid out in this book, you will see that the lower end does not provide enough protein for the two meals of whole foods needed for muscle optimization.

If you are more physically active, older, or dealing with malnutrition, acute injury, or chronic injury, 1.6 to 2.2 g/kg (0.7 to 1.0 g/lb) of protein is likely a better target range. Based on both the PROT-AGE Study group position statement and my clinical experience, these higher numbers offer more protection.[7]

However you slice it, my belief remains firm that the minimum amount of protein any adult should consume is 100 grams per day.

Note: You can find the recipes and nutritional info for these meals starting on page 289.

LONGEVITY

DAY 1

Meal 1   SHAKE + EGGS
580 calories, 50 g protein, 32 g carbs, 28 g fat, 8 g fiber

Meal 2   TURKEY CLUB LETTUCE WRAPS
297 calories, 24 g protein, 21 g carbs, 13 g fat, 9 g fiber

Meal 3   STEAK + VEG + RICE
547 calories, 49 g protein, 45 g carbs, 19 g fat, 14 g fiber

DAY 2

Meal 1   DENVER SCRAMBLE
539 calories, 49 g protein, 34 g carbs, 23 g fat, 7 g fiber

SHRIMP STIR-FRY
Meal 2   353 calories, 23 g protein, 18 g carbs, 21 g fat, 4 g fiber

BUFFALO CHICKEN SALAD
Meal 3   558 calories, 48 g protein, 43 g carbs, 22 g fat, 10 g fiber

DAY 3

Meal 1   CHIA PUDDING
435 calories, 48 g protein, 36 g carbs, 11 g fat, 11 g fiber

Meal 2   TURKEY CLUB LETTUCE WRAPS
297 calories, 24 g protein, 21 g carbs, 13 g fat, 9 g fiber

Meal 3   STEAK + VEG + RICE
547 calories, 49 g protein, 45 g carbs, 19 g fat, 14 g fiber

DAY 4

Meal 1   SHAKE + EGGS
580 calories, 50 g protein, 32 g carbs, 28 g fat, 8 g fiber

Meal 2   SHRIMP STIR-FRY
353 calories, 23 g protein, 18 g carbs, 21 g fat, 4 g fiber

Meal 3   TACO STUFFED PEPPERS
540 calories, 50 g protein, 49 g carbs, 16 g fat, 9 g fiber

DAY 5

Meal 1   DENVER SCRAMBLE
539 calories, 49 g protein, 34 g carbs, 23 g fat, 7 g fiber

Meal 2   TUNA + BEET SALAD
289 calories, 21 g protein, 22 g carbs, 13 g fat, 5 g fiber

Meal 3   COD WITH BAKED POTATO
612 calories, 51 g protein, 48 g carbs, 24 g fat, 7 g fiber

DAY 6

Meal 1   SHAKE + EGGS
580 calories, 50 g protein, 32 g carbs, 28 g fat, 8 g fiber

Meal 2   TUNA + BEET SALAD
289 calories, 21 g protein, 22 g carbs, 13 g fat, 5 g fiber

Meal 3   TACO STUFFED PEPPERS
540 calories, 50 g protein, 49 g carbs, 16 g fat, 9 g fiber

DAY 7

Meal 1   DENVER SCRAMBLE
539 calories, 49 g protein, 34 g carbs, 23 g fat, 7 g fiber

Meal 2   TURKEY CLUB LETTUCE WRAPS
297 calories, 24 g protein, 21 g carbs, 13 g fat, 9 g fiber

Meal 3   COD WITH BAKED POTATO
612 calories, 51 g protein, 48 g carbs, 24 g fat, 7 g fiber

2. OPTIMIZE QUALITY WEIGHT LOSS

Nearly 75 percent of American adults are overweight, and more than 40 percent are clinically obese. If you're ten or more pounds away from your goal weight, it's time to rebalance your dietary protein, carbohydrates, and fats. Calories count, but without making the correct choices between protein and carbohydrates, you'll be fighting a losing battle—a battle of the bulge.

Optimize Quality Weight Loss Plan Details:

■ Three meals plus one optional snack per day.

■ Even distribution of protein and carbohydrates in each meal.

■ First meal is a protein shake for calorie control.

■ If your goal is to lose ten pounds or less (or if you're a female with ≤ 28% body fat, or a male with ≤ 22% body fat), reduce your calories 10 to 20 percent below maintenance.

■ If your goal is to lose more than ten pounds, decrease your calories by 20 to 30 percent below maintenance.

PROTEIN: When you're reducing total calories, increasing your protein intake (the target is 0.8 to 1.1 grams per pound of ideal body weight) helps you retain lean body mass.[8]

■ The lower your calories, the higher your protein percentage should be.

■ To protect muscle, target your protein at 1 gram per pound of ideal body weight or potentially higher, depending on your training status.

CARBS: Start carbs on the lower side, given our goal to maintain muscle and focus on quality weight loss. If you are sedentary or have abnormal blood markers such as elevated blood sugar, insulin, or triglycerides, I suggest starting at 30 grams of carbohydrates per meal.

FAT: 0.7 to 2.2 g/kg (0.32 to 1.0 g/lb). The remainder of your calories can be dedicated to fats. If you hit a weight-loss plateau, we will reduce fat calories first.

During the first two weeks of the Optimizing Quality Weight Loss track, you should lose between two and four pounds, depending on how much weight you have to lose. You might feel hungry, but you'll be motivated by seeing the scale move. Expect a two-week adjustment period during which you must manage expectations. There is no free lunch.

Our goal here is to create slow, controlled changes in body composition. These minimize stress on the body and likely help with muscle retention. There is a lot to be learned from the world of natural bodybuilding and the research of Dr. Eric Helms. The interface between natural bodybuilding and body recomposition pushes people toward health. To maximize muscle retention, set caloric intake at a level that results in body-weight losses of approximately 0.5 to 1 percent per week.[9]

To determine your calories, we need to recognize that the tissue lost during an energy deficit is influenced by the size of the energy deficit.[10] While greater deficits yield faster weight loss, a percentage of that weight loss will come from lean body mass. Slow and steady is the way to go.

WEIGHT LOSS

DAY 1

Meal 1   PROTEIN SHAKE
           421 calories, 38 g protein, 29 g carbs, 17 g fat, 4 g fiber

Meal 2   GREEN GODDESS COBB SALAD
           422 calories, 36 g protein, 29 g carbs, 18 g fat, 9 g fiber

Meal 3   BURGER + RICE
           498 calories, 47 g protein, 29 g carbs, 21 g fat, 7 g fiber

DAY 2

Meal 1   BURGER + EGGS
           417 calories, 38 g protein, 28 g carbs, 17 g fat, 6 g fiber

Meal 2   SHRIMP STIR-FRY
            386 calories, 30 g protein, 26 g carbs, 18 g fat, 4 g fiber

Meal 3   BUFFALO CHICKEN SALAD
            433 calories, 39 g protein, 30 g carbs, 17 g fat, 8 g fiber

DAY 3

Meal 1   CHIA PUDDING
            382 calories, 42 g protein, 31 g carbs, 10 g fat, 10 g fiber

Meal 2   GREEN GODDESS COBB SALAD
            422 calories, 36 g protein, 29 g carbs, 18 g fat, 9 g fiber

Meal 3   SHRIMP STIR-FRY
            465 calories, 43 g protein, 26 g carbs, 21 g fat, 4 g fiber

DAY 4

Meal 1   PROTEIN SHAKE
            421 calories, 38 g protein, 29 g carbs, 17 g fat, 4 g fiber

Meal 2   BURGER + RICE
            421 calories, 29 g protein, 29 g carbs, 21 g fat, 6 g fiber

Meal 3   PORK + SWEET POTATOES
            462 calories, 39 g protein, 27 g carbs, 22 g fat, 5 g fiber

DAY 5

Meal 1   CHIA PUDDING
            382 calories, 42 g protein, 31 g carbs, 10 g fat, 10 g fiber

Meal 2   PORK + SWEET POTATOES
            393 calories, 33 g protein, 27 g carbs, 17 g fat, 5 g fiber

Meal 3   SALMON + BEET SALAD
            502 calories, 42 g protein, 34 g carbs, 22 g fat, 19 g fiber

DAY 6

Meal 1   BURGER + EGGS
            417 calories, 38 g protein, 28 g carbs, 17 g fat, 6 g fiber

Meal 2   TUNA + BEET SALAD
            393 calories, 26 g protein, 25 g carbs, 21 g fat, 6 g fiber

Meal 3   STEAK + GREEN BEANS
            494 calories, 43 g protein, 31 g carbs, 22 g fat, 9 g fiber

DAY 7

Meal 1   PROTEIN SHAKE
            421 calories, 38 g protein, 29 g carbs, 17 g fat, 4 g fiber

Meal 2   STEAK + GREEN BEANS
            494 calories, 43 g protein, 31 g carbs, 22 g fat, 9 g fiber

Meal 3   BUFFALO CHICKEN SALAD
            433 calories, 39 g protein, 30 g carbs, 17 g fat, 8 g fiber

3. OPTIMIZE MUSCLE

Many adults need to gain muscle. Some individuals desire the additional strength or improved physical appearance, but virtually every adult would benefit from more power, more stability, and a healthier metabolism. Muscle gain (hypertrophy) requires *both* resistance exercise training and optimizing protein intake. Protein alone will not add muscle, and inadequate protein consumption will minimize or prevent training gains. (Learn how to plan the perfect training schedule for your body type and goals on page 229.) I suggest four meals per day to allow for nutrient distribution and protein pacing. This will ensure that you reach your necessary protein threshold for muscle growth and allow you to pace the stimulation of muscle.

- Eat every three to four hours to hit your protein and total calorie intake.[11]
- Eat your target level of carbs before and after your workouts,[12] then balance the rest throughout the day. Choose options with a lower carb-to-fiber ratio such as broccoli or high-fiber oatmeal, one to two hours prior to exercise. Data show that a high insulin response at the beginning of exercise decreases total output,

power, and endurance. Consume the highest carb-to-fiber-ratio foods, such as a banana, post-exercise, especially if you have a short window until the next time you must perform.

■ Eat your lowest-fat meals before and after you train. Your body will not utilize fat for fuel quickly post-consumption, and fat slows down digestion and gastric emptying, which could lead to feeling bloated during exercise.

■ Most importantly, meet your total protein and calorie needs.

■ I recommend supplementation with creatine and fish oil.

■ Finish the protein on your plate before you move to the other foods. If you wind up struggling to finish it all, it's best that you've prioritized eating the protein first to hit the most important macronutrient for muscle health.

■ Train consistently and make steady progress with your workout plan to ensure muscle growth. Exercise is a nonnegotiable element of all my plans, but the Optimize Muscle Plan cannot work without targeted hypertrophy (muscle-growing) resistance training.

■ Carve out time for rest and recovery. Prioritize sleep, as this is when the body grows and repairs. Nearly one-third of Americans older than eighteen fail to get the recommended seven to nine hours of sleep. Chronic lack of sleep disrupts skeletal muscle and glucose levels, as well as our endocrine systems and hormones, predisposing us to health issues that include obesity, insulin resistance, and type 2 diabetes.

■ Because you will be eating more, prepping all your foods on a Sunday or ordering in bulk from a meal-prep service such as ICON Meals will help you keep up with your macro requirements.

■ Monitor your body changes in a consistent manner with either the InBody analyzer or a repeated body-composition DEXA scan to track muscle gain.

SLEEP

Studies show that disturbed sleep decreases rates of muscle-protein synthesis in healthy adult males and, over time, can result in loss of lean mass and reductions in muscle strength and functional outcomes.[13]

Both short-term (twenty-four hours of sleep deprivation) and long-term (five nights of sleep restriction) sleep disturbances cause disruption in circadian rhythms and decrease muscle-protein synthesis rates. However, implementing high-intensity interval training during periods of sleep restriction has been shown to preserve the rates of muscle-protein synthesis. In other words, exercise can mitigate some of the negative effects of reduced sleep patterns on muscle-protein synthesis rates.

- Log your strength and performance metrics, reassessing your progress every six to eight weeks. Has your performance improved? Has your strength increased? Although this is not primarily a strength program, the more skilled you become, the more effort it will take to stimulate your body. That's why regular reassessment is key.
- One final thought here. Have fun! Consider this not as a rigid routine but as a fun and exciting journey that will increase your organ of longevity.

OPTIMIZE MUSCLE PLAN DETAILS

The major drivers: sufficient energy, amino acids, resistance-training stimulus.

- Four meals per day, each containing 40 to 60 grams of protein.
- Protein: 1.0 to 1.2 grams of protein per pound of ideal body weight.
- 10 to 20 percent calorie surplus, prioritizing protein.

- Carbs: 1.4 to 3.6 grams per pound of total body weight.[14]
- Fat: 0.7 to 2.2 g/kg (.32 to 1.0 g/lb). If you prefer carb-rich over fat-rich foods, then favor the lower end of the fat calories range.

This is my highest-calorie plan, with a calorie surplus of 10 to 20 percent if you're well trained or 20 to 30 percent if you're just starting resistance training to build muscle mass. Consuming extra calories can lead to excess body fat. It's critical to track body-fat gain, which will dictate calorie surplus. Striking the right balance in body composition will take some trial and error.

MUSCLE

DAY 1

Meal 1   SHAKE + EGGS
536 calories, 49 g protein, 22 g carbs, 28 g fat, 6 g fiber

Meal 2   SALMON + BEET SALAD + RICE
470 calories, 45 g protein, 23 g carbs, 22 g fat, 3 g fiber

Meal 3   ROAST BEEF LETTUCE WRAPS
478 calories, 51 g protein, 46 g carbs, 10 g fat, 12 g fiber

Meal 4   PORK CHOP + VEG
637 calories, 52 g protein, 42 g carbs, 29 g fat, 11 g fiber

DAY 2

Meal 1   CHIA PUDDING
390 calories, 49 g protein, 26 g carbs, 10 g fat, 9 g fiber

Meal 2   SHRIMP STIR-FRY
538 calories, 49 g protein, 27 g carbs, 26 g fat, 4 g fiber

Meal 3   PORK CHOP + VEG
637 calories, 52 g protein, 42 g carbs, 29 g fat, 11 g fiber

Meal 4   BUFFALO CHICKEN SALAD
623 calories, 56 g protein, 49 g carbs, 23 g fat, 11 g fiber

DAY 3

Meal 1   SHAKE + EGGS
536 calories, 49 g protein, 22 g carbs, 28 g fat, 6 g fiber

Meal 2   SALMON + BEET SALAD + RICE
470 calories, 45 g protein, 23 g carbs, 22 g fat, 3 g fiber

Meal 3   ROAST BEEF LETTUCE WRAPS
478 calories, 51 g protein, 46 g carbs, 10 g fat, 12 g fiber

Meal 4   PORK LOIN + VEG
586 calories, 45 g protein, 43 g carbs, 26 g fat, 17 g fiber

DAY 4

Meal 1   DENVER SCRAMBLE
535 calories, 48 g protein, 34 g carbs, 23 g fat, 7 g fiber

Meal 2   "SPAGHETTI" WITH MEAT SAUCE
508 calories, 49 g protein, 24 g carbs, 24 g fat, 5 g fiber

Meal 3   BUFFALO CHICKEN SALAD
623 calories, 56 g protein, 49 g carbs, 23 g fat, 11 g fiber

Meal 4   PORK LOIN + VEG
586 calories, 45 g protein, 43 g carbs, 26 g fat, 17 g fiber

DAY 5

Meal 1   CHIA PUDDING
390 calories, 49 g protein, 26 g carbs, 10 g fat, 9 g fiber

Meal 2   SHRIMP STIR-FRY
538 calories, 49 g protein, 27 g carbs, 26 g fat, 4 g fiber

Meal 3   PORK LOIN + VEG
586 calories, 45 g protein, 43 g carbs, 26 g fat, 17 g fiber

Meal 4   BURGER SALAD
592 calories, 49 g protein, 45 g carbs, 24 g fat, 10 g fiber

DAY 6

Meal 1   SHAKE + EGGS
          536 calories, 49 g protein, 22g carbs, 28 g fat, 6 g fiber

Meal 2   "SPAGHETTI" WITH MEAT SAUCE
          508 calories, 49 g protein, 24 g carbs, 24 g fat, 5 g fiber

Meal 3   TUNA MELT
          664 calories, 53 g protein, 50 g carbs, 28 g fat, 12 g fiber

Meal 4   BURGER SALAD
          592 calories, 49 g protein, 45 g carbs, 24 g fat, 10 g fiber

DAY 7

Meal 1   DENVER SCRAMBLE
          535 calories, 48 g protein, 34 g carbs, 23 g fat, 7 g fiber

Meal 2   ROAST BEEF LETTUCE WRAPS
          467 calories, 50 g protein, 24 g carbs, 19 g fat, 9 g fiber

Meal 3   COD WITH BAKED POTATO
          612 calories, 51 g protein, 48 g carbs, 24 g fat, 7 g fiber

Meal 4   BUFFALO CHICKEN SALAD
          623 calories, 56 g protein, 49 g carbs, 23 g fat, 11 g fiber

NEED A TREAT? TRY COCONUT MILK "ICE CREAM"

1 banana, sliced and frozen
1 cup pineapple chunks, frozen
¼ cup canned coconut milk

1. Place the banana, pineapple, and coconut milk in a food processor and blend.
2. Occasionally scrape down the sides and continue to blend until smooth, about 3 minutes.
3. Scoop into a bowl and enjoy immediately as soft serve, or for firmer ice cream, place in an airtight, freezer-safe container and freeze for at least 1 hour before scooping.

If you'd like more recipe options with at least 30 grams of protein, go to www.drgabriellelyon.com/30gs-recipes/ and sign up for "30gs Recipes." My team and I will send you weekly recipes to remove the guesswork about what to put on your plate.

TRY THIS: CARNIVORE RESET

The carnivore reset is a great way to chalk up an early win. You might be familiar with plant-based elimination diets. Well, this is an animal-based elimination diet. It entails very high animal-product intake with very low vegetable intake. Follow this protocol for two to four weeks. Not only do many people feel remarkably better after this protocol, but their blood metrics also reflect positive changes. My carnivore reset recommendation is reminiscent of the **Protein-Sparing Modified Fast Program at Cleveland Clinic**. At present, this is not an "evidence-based plan" but rather what I have used in my clinic with great success over the years.

My carnivore reset includes:

Eggs, meat, fish, and a first-meal protein shake for calorie control. The shake contains 50 g whey or rice/pea blend protein, 1 scoop of green or red powder for phytonutrients (e.g., prebiotic fibers and polyphenols, vitamin C, lutein), 1 tablespoon of medium-chain triglyceride powder, and almond milk or water. (If your body can't tolerate dairy, you can replace the whey powder with 1.5 scoops of beef protein plus ½ scoop [3 grams] of leucine powder to mimic the high leucine of dairy protein.)

In this protocol, individuals can consume any animal products except dairy (outside of a protein powder), as these can cause inflammation, constipation, or bloating. Acceptable plant foods include cilantro, parsley, scallions, and jalapeños.

While the focus of this reset isn't calorie control, men can target consuming 1,800 to 1,900 calories a day, while women can target 1,500 to 1,600 calories during this period.

This low-volume, nutrient-dense, flavor-packed protocol is an excellent way to jump-start weight loss, crush cravings, and build momentum toward your optimized lifestyle.

EVENING RITUAL

Ask yourself these questions:

1. Am I proud of the choices I made today?

2. Did I exhibit the characteristics that are worthy of the person I strive to become?

3. What is one thing that I can do better tomorrow?

4. How can I prepare myself to prevent repeating any unhealthy behaviors that I know I'll confront in the future? (For example, say every time you go to the kitchen at ten o'clock at night, you wind up eating a cookie. Think ahead. There's no surprise here. Prepare for the next time this impulse occurs, dream up an alternative outcome, then bring that to life.)

5. Given tomorrow's schedule, what is my strategy for making the choices that will help me stick with my plan?

MINDSET RESET

ERECTING GUARDRAILS FOR ACCOUNTABILITY

My goal is to help you develop scaffolding so stable it will keep you from falling off your goal wagon no matter what obstacles arise. This requires shoring up the underlying operating system that determines how you process, execute, and internalize your experiences. How do you gauge your own wellness? How do you perceive your relationship with your physician? How do you understand integrity and your responsibilities to yourself? Bringing this underlying system into conscious awareness is critical to upgrading and optimizing it. How you process the experience will determine the outcome.

Next, make a clear, concrete plan with measurable objectives. Why is a plan so important?

1. A plan erects guardrails for your integrity and frees your mind to focus on other things. You won't need to constantly think *What should I eat?* or *How should I train?* because you'll already know the answers.
2. A plan removes all the what-ifs—the questions that prevent you from keeping consistent—and eliminates any opportunity for negotiation about meals or training.

Reining in your mind and its internal narratives will immediately put you on the road to success. Practicing mental discipline will help you regulate your emotions and beliefs. This means you must first catch and bring to awareness any repetitive deadbeat thoughts keeping you from reaching your dreams.

Here's an example from my own life. When I found my-self parenting a toddler while pregnant, I could have focused on the voice that told me I was too emotional and anxious to train or complete my work. Instead, I recognized those thoughts as dream blockers. Such thoughts can include anything cloaked in heightened anxiety or emotion. Even being hard on yourself can serve as distraction.

By upgrading your inner operating system and erecting a solid plan, you can give up excesses (substances/time wasters/ negative emotional attributes), including too much of the fol-lowing:

- Alcohol
- Stimulants
- Sugar
- Bread
- TV/social media
- Negativity
- Dishonesty
- Social outings
- Calls/texts

. . . all of which can serve as enticing distractions.

Keep your world small—at least at first. Hold yourself ac-countable. Success comes from each small execution of the task at hand.

8.

~~~~~~~~~~

Baseline Assessment:
Where Are You?

Knowing where you are is critical to getting where you're going. Ask yourself: *What are my goals, and how can I reach them?* Then reverse engineer the action steps that will ensure success. Making lasting fat-loss changes and maximizing the muscle that supports longevity must begin with a careful self-assessment.

A look at numbers from your annual physical exam can reveal a lot about your health risks and offer clues about how to optimize your diet. Your height, weight, waist circumference, blood triglycerides, and fasting blood sugar all help define your needs and goals for nutrition success. I strongly advise that you work with a dietitian and a fitness professional to help guide, track, and hone your decision-making around the therapeutic use of both diet and physical training. Arming yourself with an expanded list of your metrics is a great first step.

BLOOD PRESSURE

High blood pressure (hypertension) is, hands down, the most common—and preventable!—risk factor for early heart disease. High-blood-pressure risk outweighs high cholesterol, diabetes, and even cigarette smoking.

But often, unfortunately, these other risk factors coexist with hypertension, compounding overall risk. An unhealthy diet, physical inactivity, and being overweight or obese also raise cardiovascular disease risk.

When evaluating blood-pressure health, I follow the standards established by the American Heart Association and the American College of Cardiology in 2017:

- Normal = less than 120 (systolic) *and* less than 80 (diastolic)
- Elevated = 120–129 *and* less than 80
- High blood pressure stage 1 = 130–139 *or* 80–89
- High blood pressure stage 2 = 140 or higher *or* 90 or higher
- Hypertensive crisis (call your doctor immediately!) = higher than 180 *and/or* higher than 120

WAIST CIRCUMFERENCE AND WAIST-TO-HEIGHT RATIO

Waist circumference (WC) is a quick, easy way to assess your own personal cardiovascular risk. Unlike the subcutaneous fat that we can see under our skin, visceral fat is hard to measure without imaging. That's why we use WC as a proxy; this measurement paints a clearer picture of health than body mass index (BMI) because it identifies the location of the fat.

So what does fat around your middle have to do with health? Waist circumference is strongly associated with all-cause mortality; the wider it is, the greater your chance of death from any cause. According to the National Heart, Lung, and Blood Institute, if most of your fat is around your waist rather than your hips, you're at a higher risk for heart disease and type 2 diabetes.[1] Your risk increases further with a waist size that is greater than 35 inches (88 centimeters) for women or greater than 40 inches (102 centimeters) for men.[2] Too much midsection fat is associated with higher amounts of visceral fat—the fat surrounding your organs, called visceral adiposity—that then correlates with high blood-fat levels, high blood pressure, and diabetes as well as inflammation.[3]

During my fellowship, we frequently used waist circumference to monitor and assess risk, not only for cardiovascular and metabolic function but also to predict cognitive impairment later in life.[4] However, there is now evidence suggesting that, in adults, waist-to-height ratio may be better than both BMI and waist circumference alone at identifying early risk for many of the diseases discussed in this book.[5]

To correctly calculate your waist circumference, wrap a tape measure around your midsection, just above your hip bones. Do this while standing, just after you exhale. (For a video showing how to take an accurate measurement, head to my YouTube channel, https://www.youtube.com/@DrGabrielleLyon.) Ideally, your waist circumference should total less than half your height.

A **waist-to-height ratio** (**WHtR**) above 0.5 identifies people with "early health risks" associated with central obesity.[6] To determine your WHtR, divide your waist circumference by your height, both measured in the same units. For example, if you stand 5 feet 7 inches tall, that equals 67 inches. If your waist is 36 inches around, you would divide 67 by 36 to get 0.53. To protect both mental and physical health, your goal should be to keep your waist circumference to less than half of your height, ideally a WHtR of less than 0.5.

PERCENT BODY FAT

Health professionals typically use BMI thresholds, as established by the WHO, to diagnose overweight and obesity. But as you've just seen, these numbers tell us very little about actual body composition. More instructive is gauging body-fat percentage, although determining the exact numbers takes a bit of effort.

Generally speaking, men with body fat greater than or equal to 25 percent are considered obese. For women, obesity begins at 35 percent.[7] But instead of using this binary categorization, we should be identifying and targeting an *ideal* body-fat percentage. This would promote true health improvements.

MUSCLE MASS

Looking at muscle-mass measurements alone is not enough to determine the health of your skeletal muscle or your risk for sarcopenia. **Skeletal-muscle mass needs to be assessed in combination with strength measures.** Skeletal-muscle mass is the largest component of fat-free body mass, called lean body mass. This term describes the fat-free and bone-free elements of your body, including muscle, skin, tendons, and connective tissues.[8]

The science is abundantly clear that increased healthy muscle mass leads to improved health. So how do we measure muscle mass, specifically? In short, it's possible but requires equipment. Either a DEXA (Dual-Energy X-ray Absorptiometry) whole-body composition scan or bioelectrical impedance analysis (BIA) can assess appendicular skeletal-muscle mass (ASMM), which is the mass of skeletal muscle in your extremities—basically, your legs and arms—that provides a critical data point for health assessment. The most common BIA devices are the professional-grade InBody 720 (a stationary device used to assess body composition) and the portable, more affordable version, called the InBody H20N (available at inbodyusa.com).

A simple, if a bit pricey, way to get the "gold standard" body-composition testing using X-ray technology is through a place like DEXA Scan. (Find a nearby location at dexascan.com.) Lying on the scanning bed for less than ten minutes can reveal how lean muscle, fat, water, and bone are distributed within your body.

If neither of those options works for you, a home scale can still be helpful, though slightly less accurate. Body composition is affected by hydration level and menstrual cycle, and your weight can fluctuate throughout the day. But taking measurements at the same time daily will provide the most accurate results.

ASSESSMENT TOOLS AND TRACKING SUPPLIES

BODY COMPOSITION

- **InBody H20N Whole Body Composition** (weight range 22 lb–330 lb) at-home scale, $279.20.
- **Tape measure**, price varies.
- **Samsung Galaxy Watch 4**, $279.99.

OVERALL HEALTH

- **Glucose monitor, Nutrisense**, 1-, 3-, 6-, and 12-month programs ranging from $199 to $350 per month.
- **Apple Watch**, starts at $399.
- **Grip strength**, e.g., CAMRY Digital Hand Dynamometer, $30.

NUTRITIONAL TRACKING

- **Food scale**, e.g., Etekcity Food Scale, $14.
- **Cronometer**, food-tracking app (free version available).

Although different methods of measuring muscle mass have slight differences in accuracy, a DEXA scan is generally considered the most accurate of available practical options. (MRI and CT scans would, of course, offer definitive numbers, but these diagnostics result in too much radiation for casual use.)

However it's done, assessing an individual's ASMM offers a simple, effective gauge of overall health and risk of getting or dying from disease (morbidity/mortality). In the same way that we can assess muscle mass to identify sarcopenia, we should use this approach more broadly to identify a range of muscle-mass levels across ages and athletic body types. Unfortunately, no universal standard among physicians or academics currently exists for optimal levels, only levels that focus on disease. Therefore, my recommendation is to build and maintain as much healthy muscle as you can. Meanwhile, check out this pioneering approach to gauging skeletal muscle. I created the chart below with Dr. Alexis Cowan, a highly trained Princeton researcher, using data from some of the country's best labs.[9] It may look complicated, but it's simple.

KEY: Sarcopenia is defined as appendicular skeletal muscle mass of less than 7.0 kg/m2 for men and less than 5.4 kg/m2 for women (as measured by DEXA)

Demographic	DEXA Scan skeletal muscle (kg/m²)	InBody H20N skeletal muscle (kg/m²)	InBody 720 skeletal muscle (kg/m²)
Average adult male (< 65)	8.6	9.5	10.5
Average adult female (< 65)	7.3	7.3	10.6
Athletic male	10.2	11.7	13.0
Athletic female	8.0	8.6	11.4
Mature male (65+)	7.7	8.1	8.7
Mature female (65+)	5.9	5.3	7.8
Under-muscled male (sarcopenic)	7.0	7.2	7.4
Under-muscled female (sarcopenic)	5.4	4.6	6.9

Body composition is reported in the standard units of kilograms of muscle divided by height in meters squared. It is divided into average (meaning of normal health), athletic, mature (65+), and sarcopenic (not enough muscle).

If you don't have access to measure your muscle mass with a DEXA scan or the InBody scale, please take this muscle health quiz:

DETERMINING YOUR MUSCLE HEALTH

GENERAL HEALTH

Age: ❏ < 45 (1)   ❏ 45–65 (0)   ❏ > 65 years (-2)

Gender: ❏ M or ❏ F

Weight (pounds): _____

Height (inches): _____

BMI: ❏ > 35 (–2)   ❏ 28–35 (–1)   ❏ < 28 (+1)

FITNESS

What is your athletic type?

❏ Lifelong athlete (1)
❏ Fitness junkie (2)
❏ Weekend warrior (occasionally work out) (0)
❏ Couch potato (–2)

Resistance exercise (days per week spending at least 45 minutes with weights or yoga training):

❏ 0 days (0)
❏ 1 (1)
❏ 2–3 (3)
❏ > 3 (5)

Aerobic exercise (days per week spending at least 45 minutes with running, elliptical, swimming, biking, or singles tennis; activities that increase both breathing and heart rate):

❑ 0 days (0)

❑ 1 (1)

❑ 2–3 (2)

❑ > 3 (3)

NUTRITION

Indicate the amount of each of the following that you consumed during the past 7 days to help estimate your daily protein intake for the Protein Scoring section below.

Eggs: _____

Milk or yogurt (glass or cup servings; indicate servings/week): _____

Meats (beef, pork, chicken, or fish; serving is 4 ounces): _____

Beans or lentils (serving is 1 cup): _____

PROTEIN SCORING

> 140 g/day (5)

110–139 (3)

90–110 (2)

75–90 (0)

< 75 (–1)

Note: We estimate 1 egg = 6 g protein; milk or yogurt = 8 g; meats (4 ounces) = 28 g; beans = 12 g. We also assume everyone gets about 25 g/day of protein from grains. From these estimates and body weight, we would set a "healthy muscle threshold" of 1.2–1.5g/kg/day.

MUSCLE AGE (Based on Total Scores Above)

10 or higher: Young and thriving

6–9: Could use some work

5 or less: Need a muscle makeover

LAB WORK: THE INSIDE STORY

To map any journey forward, we need to know where we're standing. So let's dig in to help you discover more about your baseline. **Blood markers can reveal health information that you can improve directly—through lifestyle changes alone.** Did you know you can order your own custom lab work for a more detailed picture of your health? I will guide you through exactly which panels to request, and when, based on the information each specific result can provide. I'll also teach you how to examine your own metrics, establish reasonable targets for improved health, and translate those targets into achievable, measurable goals.

Plan to get a blood draw at your physician's office or through a direct-to-consumer lab. (I recommend InsideTracker, at store.inside tracker.com, and you can use the code DRLYON for a discount.) The resulting lab work will provide objective measurements of critical systems. Think of yourself as the pilot, your body as the plane, and your blood markers as the gauges in a cockpit that inform the decisions that ensure a successful flight.

Lab work serves as a foundational element of my clinical practice, showing my patients where they're starting from, pointing them toward progress and, later, measuring their successes. **Here, for this book, I've restricted my typical lab orders strictly to variables that you can impact directly, on your own, through diet and exercise.** Each of these benchmarks improves when you gain muscle and lose fat. In addition, since skeletal muscle is a primary regulator of both carbohydrates and fats, your muscle-health measurements will impact the metabolism of your diet.[10] Future directions will likely include measuring myokines post-exercise to determine, in part, the effectiveness of our workouts so we can fine-tune exercise as a prescription.

LIPID REGULATION

First, let's talk lipids. Examination of lipid regulation involves two domains, dietary and metabolic, indicating what you eat and how your body uses these fats. Your typical annual workup likely includes a lipid panel that assesses your total cholesterol, HDL cholesterol, LDL cholesterol (calculated or direct measurement), and triglycerides. These important measures help gauge your risk of heart disease—a risk that increases when elevated levels of fats circulate in the bloodstream. While cholesterol is an essential ingredient for building healthy cells, too much can lead to fatty-deposit buildup that can obstruct blood flow through your arteries. High triglycerides cause similar problems.

Triglycerides

Each time you eat more calories than you use right away, the body converts the remainder into triglycerides (TG). TGs represent the storage form of fatty acids within the cells and blood, and they serve as a major transport form of fat to support tissue energy production. Following a meal in healthy individuals, triglyceride levels climb as dietary fat is transported in the bloodstream by particles known as lipoproteins. The lipoproteins primarily deliver these triglycerides to adipose tissue for storage, while some will also be used to support the functionality of tissues like the heart. Triglycerides are lower in the fasted than in the fed state, and free fatty acids emerge as a major source of fat to fuel tissue energy needs. However, both triglycerides and free fatty acids serve as important sources of fat-derived energy in the fasted state.

TG stored in and around muscle instead of adipose tissue that remains there in a stagnant pool indicates impaired fat oxidation capacity in muscle: a hallmark of insulin resistance. In this scenario, your body's ability to manage extra calories becomes more and more dysfunctional over time as muscular fat accumulates.

Regularly consuming more calories than you burn, particularly from high-carbohydrate foods, can lead to elevated TG levels that increase your risk of heart attack, stroke, pancreatitis, and nonalcoholic fatty liver disease. High TG is a signal indicating excess energy, that you are taking in more than you are expending. You have likely heard of nonalcoholic fatty liver disease, but the same thing happens in muscle. According to guidelines from the National Cholesterol Education Program's Adult Treatment Panel III (ATP III), TG levels, measured in the blood after a twelve-hour fast, are classified as normal at less than 150 mg/dL, as borderline high at 150 to 199 mg/dL, as high at 200 to 499 mg/dL, or as very high at greater than or equal to 500 mg/dL. However, the recent American Heart Association scientific statement on TG notes that low fasting triglyceride levels (i.e., less than 100 mg/dL) are commonly found in countries at relatively low coronary artery disease risk compared with the US. **I recommend an optimal fasting TG level of less than 100 mg/dL and an optimal nonfasting TG level of less than 150 mg/dL.**

ACTION ITEM ➤ Dietary TG can show an increase four hours after eating. More consistent change shows over weeks and days. I recommend retesting after two to three months of consistent lifestyle change.

HDL Cholesterol

HDL cholesterol is yet another marker that's directly improved by exercise. HDL helps clear other cholesterol from the bloodstream, and higher levels are associated with decreased risk of heart disease. Although HDL is commonly referred to as the "good cholesterol," the real story is a bit more complicated. HDL has many roles, and there are no lab markers that show you how HDL is acting in the system. For HDL to have health benefits, it needs to be functional. In some cases, high inflammation can damage HDL, causing your body to keep making more as replacement. In this scenario, more is not better. Exercise is one of the best ways to increase healthy HDL cholesterol. Adding more omega-3s to your diet can also help.

People with obesity, elevated blood pressure, and high blood-sugar levels typically have lower levels of HDL. Increasing physical activity can help raise their HDL levels, with benefits visible after just sixty minutes of moderate aerobic exercise weekly. High-intensity interval training (HIIT) seems to have the biggest impact on HDL and functionality.

What are optimal levels of HDL cholesterol?

	At risk	Healthy
Men	Less than 40 mg/dL	60 mg/dL or above
Women	Less than 50 mg/dL	60 mg/dL or above[11]

ACTION ITEM ➤ Retest HDL levels after two to three months of consistent lifestyle change.

LDL Cholesterol

Although LDL cholesterol is not as clinically relevant as we once thought, it remains a hot topic of conversation. The American Heart Association blames high LDL cholesterol in most people on an unhealthy lifestyle,[12] but genetic inheritance is a significant cause of increased levels. Moderate exercise can lower LDL cholesterol by 10 to 15 percent. Aerobic physical activity at or above the minimum threshold of around 1,200 kcal weekly may be an effective strategy for managing lipid profiles and reducing cardiovascular disease risk.[13] The literature, however, shows tremendous variability of impact. For some, diet modification can change LDL cholesterol levels as much as 17 to 25 percent.[14] In my clinical practice, however, I've seen that many people are unable to lower their LDL cholesterol levels through dietary change by any more than 10 percent.

Instead, a genetic set point typically drives increased LDL cholesterol. Research suggests that heritability explains 40 to 50 percent of plasma LDL levels.[15] This becomes an important counterpoint to the widespread recommendations that a heart-healthy diet requires eating less saturated fat, particularly red meat. I argue that if you do not have genetic issues with LDL cholesterol and you keep your calories controlled, then saturated fat will not cause problems. For our purposes, when it comes to LDL cholesterol, we will maintain focus on the average person instead of those with genetic challenges.

How can you tell if you have a genetic issue or if diet and exercise will help? If you have strong family history of early cardiovascular disease with elevated cholesterol (higher than 300) and LDL (higher than 190), genetics may be the issue. If you had "normal" lipids at some point and then followed a keto diet or some other lifestyle intervention and numbers skyrocketed, then even with a genetic component in the equation, lifestyle choices can likely help reduce your numbers. Reaching an LDL level considered "normal" could require a multifaceted approach depending on primary versus secondary prevention methods.

Primary prevention: If your LDL levels are lower than 190 mg/dL, work with your physician or cardiologist to determine your risk factors.

Secondary prevention: If your LDL is higher than 190 mg/dL, your levels are most likely genetically driven and may require pharmaceutical intervention. This is because dietary changes may aid in lowering the number, but your body will eventually return to the baseline that is genetically set.

ACTION ITEM ➤ Test LDL levels yearly with your annual blood panels.

APOLIPOPROTEIN B

HDL and LDL are commonly referred to in conversations about heart health. But have you heard of this other indicator, apolipoprotein B (apo-B)? Measuring apo-B, the protein component of LDL, homes in specifically on the number of LDL particles (LDL-P) so we can more accurately gauge heart health.

I liken LDL-P to cargo ships hauling around LDL of various sizes. Too many small ships (i.e., small LDL particles) can gum up your waterways (arteries)—increasing the probability that they become wedged in the arterial wall. It's important to note that particle size is tightly linked with insulin sensitivity, with more small particles indicating insulin resistance. Furthermore, as LDL particle size decreases, the *total* number of LDL particles tends to increase. The more LDL particles you have in your bloodstream, the greater the chances that these particles will bang up against artery walls. This is why, compared to large LDL particles, small LDL particles are associated with higher risk of cardiovascular disease.

The protein apo-B helps carry fat, cholesterol, and phospholipids throughout your body. Careful examination of existing literature reveals apo-B as a far better metric for gauging cardiovascular health than LDL cholesterol. Each LDL-P contains one molecule of apo-B. A higher apo-B level means a higher LDL-P level, which suggests greater cardiac risk. **Given all this, a good target level for your apo-B is less than 80 mg/dL, with an ideal level of 60 mg/dL.**

ACTION ITEM ➤ Test apo-B levels every three to six months—three months if you have elevated levels and less often if you've already hit the ideal range.

LIVER ENZYMES

Other blood markers we can use to track improved body composition are two enzymes released from the liver, alanine aminotransferase (ALT) and aspartate aminotransferase (AST). Obesity and excess weight can cause fat deposits to accumulate in the liver, leading to chronic inflammation and scarring, often without causing any noticeable symptoms. Measuring ALT and AST can not only reveal the presence of nonalcoholic fatty liver disease but also **show liver-health improvements brought about by weight loss.**[16]

Ideal ALT blood levels total less than 20 units per liter of serum for women and less than 30 units for men. I typically recommend that my patients continue to lose weight until they reach these target levels. Although studies show that liver enzymes may temporarily rise immediately following diet-induced weight loss in women, these increases, when transient, are considered benign, with no cause for alarm.[17] It's also important to note that intense exercise can also increase levels of these enzymes.

Alanine aminotransferase (ALT):[18]
- Male: 29 to 33 units/L
- Female: 19 to 25 units/L

Aspartate aminotransferase (AST):

■ Male: 10 to 40 units/L
■ Female: 9 to 32 units/L

ACTION ITEM ➤ Test ALT and AST levels every three to six months.

INFLAMMATION MARKERS

Inflammation is a recognized trigger of heart attacks, heart failure, and strokes, among other cardiovascular disease events. Emerging biomarkers of inflammation can play an important role in identifying at-risk patients, even before symptoms appear. While LDL cholesterol levels are more commonly discussed as indicators of heart health, studies suggest that serum levels of high-sensitivity C-reactive protein (hs-CRP) are a stronger predictor of cardiovascular trouble.[19] Because levels of this nonspecific, yet critical, marker of inflammation are powerful predictors of mortality overall,[20] **I recommend using hs-CRP as a general "tell" for body inflammation** because this protein reacts grossly to inflammation, facilitates damaging plaque deposits, and triggers immune responses.[21] **Ideally, this number should be less than one.** Even low-grade inflammation, indicated by just slightly elevated serum levels, can be significant. Data suggesting that low-grade inflammation and obesity make it more difficult to build muscle[22] only further emphasize how imperative it is for people in this situation to rework their body composition and gain momentum.

Tracking hs-CRP may also be a promising biomarker of visceral fat quantity and dysfunction, highlighting the type of fat that typically has very toxic effects on the body. This marker of inflammation rides along with the unhealthy muscle seen in sarcopenic obesity. Primarily produced in the liver but also in other areas in the body such as white blood cells, hs-CRP acts as the body's response to infection or inflammation. It may facilitate the interaction of immune cells such as macrophages as they bind to oxidized LDL cholesterol. As mentioned previously, the myokines produced during muscle contraction with exercise can counteract this inflammation response. Evidence suggests that, irrespective of lipid decreases, lowering hs-CRP has a positive effect on cardiovascular outcomes.[23]

ACTION ITEM ➤ Test hs-CRP every three to six months.

SUGAR REGULATION

Glucose, as discussed, is the sugar that travels through your bloodstream that is essential for proper brain, heart, and digestive function yet becomes toxic in excess. Measuring blood-glucose levels provides a clear indication of how your body is balancing food and exercise, given other physiological factors.

Glucose enters the bloodstream in three different ways: through the diet, the liver, and the kidneys. Your blood-glucose level rises when sugar from food is absorbed from the intestines after eating. It falls to its lowest between meals, after training, or following a long period without food (such as before your first daily meal). The breakdown of stored glucose (glycogen) in the liver is the second source of glucose, and the third results from gluconeogenesis, when newly created glucose gets released from the kidneys and the liver.

To lower blood-glucose levels, the body requires insulin. When blood sugar drops too low, the body will try to increase glucagon, stress hormones, cortisol, and growth hormone—all of which can help rebalance the system. Another effective way to regulate blood-glucose levels, as discussed, is through exercise, because muscle contractions use up glucose. Stored as glycogen, the glucose in muscle contributes indirectly to blood-glucose levels through a metabolite called lactate.

In today's sugar-focused, carb-crazy society, blood glucose can wind up being a double-edged sword. While our bodies require a certain amount of blood sugar in circulation, too much is toxic. It's well established that eating carbohydrates increases blood sugar more than proteins or fats. In fact, blood-sugar levels remain more stable among individuals who consume a higher-protein diet and engage in enough vigorous exercise to reach gluconeogenesis, rather than relying on food intake and liver glycogen.

Our bodies use tight regulation mechanisms to help maintain correct glucose levels, measured in millimoles of sugar per liter of blood (mmol/L). Blood sugar at baseline totals about one teaspoon of glucose at any given time. But poor lifestyle choices can throw off this delicate system, raising or lowering blood sugar to unhealthy and even dangerous levels. Hypoglycemia and hyperglycemia are two such stress states.

- Sustained levels of high blood sugar, called hyperglycemia, are a hallmark feature of type 2 diabetes.[24] Possible long-term effects include damage to organs and blood vessels, which can lead to heart attack, stroke, and other problems.
- Hypoglycemia, or low blood sugar, on the other hand, causes a variety of nervous-system problems such as weakness, light-headedness, dizziness, headaches, and irritability or confusion. A severe drop in blood glucose can cause seizures or even death.

Clearly, blood-sugar levels have a significant impact on health. That's why I incorporate regular measurement into my patient plans. One tool I recommend as part of the Lyon Protocol is a continuous glucose monitor. Available over the counter, this monitor provides real-time data that give a great picture of metabolic health. Experiment with this device to see exactly how your choices impact your metabolism.

What levels are we looking for? For someone with healthy blood-sugar regulation, blood glucose should be 140 mg/dL or less, two hours after eating. Healthy fasting glucose levels run between 70 and 99 mg/dL.

Glycated Hemoglobin A1C

The glucose bonded to hemoglobin in red blood cells, called glycated hemoglobin (HbA1C or A1C), has become the gold-standard measurement for assessing glycemic control over time. Since the average life span of red blood cells is approximately 120 days, allowing gradual accumulation of glucose over approximately three months, the results from this test represent the average glucose exposure over a three-month period.

My patients who eat a higher-protein diet tend to run a higher HbA1C as well as higher glucose, which is still within the range of normal. This occurs for two reasons. First, a portion of the amino acids in protein are converted into glucose by the liver, which increases glucose levels moderately but nowhere near as much as dietary carbohydrates do. Second, eating a balanced-macros diet maintains a more even blood-sugar level. This stable level remains within normal limits, just higher on the spectrum because my patients are able to maintain stable levels versus having the crashes that come from a more typical high-carb diet. These nuances remind us that rather than focusing simply on individual markers, we must look carefully at overall patterns.

- Normal hemoglobin A1C ranges between 4.0 and 5.6 percent.
- A level between 5.7 and 6.4 percent indicates prediabetes and a higher chance of getting diabetes.
- A level of 6.5 percent or higher means you have diabetes.

After-Meal Glucose Response

Measurement of after-meal (postprandial) glucose response reveals your body's reaction to a meal. **Normal glucose tolerance should not exceed 140 mg/dL and should return to a normal fasting blood-sugar level after a two-hour period.**

If elevated glucose following meals poses an issue, we can use training as a tool for correction. Exercise will lower blood sugar, using muscle as medicine. Using a continuous glucose monitor will allow you to gauge the effectiveness of your workouts.[25] It will also allow you to see, in real time, if an after-meal walk is sufficient to keep blood glucose in check or if you require more rigorous activity such as air squats. The goal is to be able to leverage muscle as an organ to balance the glucose system.

ACTION ITEM ➤ Test your glucose levels, specifically how often your blood sugar is elevated over a period of time, by performing a glucose tolerance test, wearing a glucose monitor, or doing a finger stick after meals.

MEDICATIONS THAT CAN CAUSE WEIGHT GAIN

❶ Steroids

❷ Antihistamines

❸ SSRIs

❹ Migraine prevention meds

❺ Insulin, glipizide, and pioglitazone

❻ Beta blockers and angiotensin-receptor blockers

❼ Birth control, particularly Depo-Provera

❽ Antipsychotics

MEDICATIONS THAT CAN NEGATIVELY IMPACT SKELETAL MUSCLE[26]

Because it makes up a large percentage of body mass, skeletal muscle is highly susceptible to the negative effects of some medications. The continuous dynamic remodeling process of muscle, with both a rich blood supply and a high tissue-turnover rate, means drugs such as the following can be myotoxic in several ways.

1. Statins
2. Sulfonylureas
3. Glinides

PHYSICAL FITNESS ASSESSMENT

It can be difficult to accurately gauge your own exercise effectiveness. Tremendous variation in focus, effort, execution, and even self-worth can muddy the waters. Still, I believe it's important to assess your physical fitness at the outset of any program. If you don't know where you are starting from, how can you know where you are going?

Food is easy to track. I can evaluate a food diary clinically, but I can never evaluate the effort you're putting into your training. Only you can know how hard you're working to realize your goals. That said, I can (and will!) help you build the structure to support your efforts. Together we'll create the environment that will see you through to attaining the extraordinary health you deserve.

Speaking of deserving . . . let's take a moment here to discuss self-worth. Far too often in my practice, I see that a self-worth deficit is the unspoken, likely unrecognized force behind a patient's hopelessness about making body-composition improvements, not to mention excuses for why they "can't" put in the effort that drives real change. Identifying the real culprit behind your resistance can help you shake free of the pessimism and devalued sense of self that keep you stuck on the hamster wheel of poor health.

MEASURING YOUR SELF-WORTH TEMPERATURE

To visualize your self-worth temperature, think of a needle on a gauge indicating the level on a scale from 0 to 100. The number on this "thermometer" will feed into your mental framework. The closer to 0, the less worthy you feel and the lower your self-worth. The higher the number, the more you value yourself and the more likely you'll be able to reach your wellness and longevity goals. This number is not a clinical assessment, of course, but the image can help identify a boost or barrier to your progress.

A SELF-WORTH TEMPERATURE QUIZ

Once you've tracked your inner monologue, identified your personal loops, and dedicated yourself to talking back to them, you've mastered the self-talk element of mental framework. With a clear understanding of the role of self-talk in our ability to achieve our goals, we can dive one layer deeper to investigate self-worth. This single factor, which I define as how you feel about yourself, will play a huge role in your ability to pass through the doors of phenomenal execution of a wellness plan.

We can gauge your self-worth temperature by tallying the answers to the following questions, scored on a scale of 1 to 5, where 1 = no, 2 = rarely (less than 20 percent of the time), 3 = occasionally (50 percent of the time), 4 = often (70 percent of the time), and 5 = always.

Do you feel worthy of having the body you desire? _____

Do you believe you can achieve this goal? _____

Do you feel worthy of having energy, enjoying the physical freedom you desire, and functioning without struggle? _____

Do you feel as if everyone has it easier and that you need to settle for the health that you currently have? _____

The answers to these questions will help you understand your baseline. Then you can get to work on elevating all these responses into the 5 zone, meaning you *always* recognize that you are worthy of the health you desire.

Everyone has a self-worth temperature that influences wellness-goal achievement. It keeps us exactly where we, deep down, feel we deserve to be. The people who succeed are those who leverage acknowledgment of their own self-worth level to mobilize into action.

And now it's time to move on to the final section of your assessment: physical performance.

PHYSICAL PERFORMANCE

Here you'll find a beginner- or intermediate-friendly assessment to help you gauge your starting point and track your improvements in four to six weeks. The goal of this assessment is to benchmark your "before" and "after" by charting a set of simple exercises that are safe for you to do without a health professional. If you're working without a partner, I recommend video-recording yourself for the first three exercises so you can view your form from an outside perspective. Put in your max effort, and don't let the first set of numbers discourage you. This is only a starting point, and with consistency, you will be amazed by the changes you'll see over the next four to six weeks!

Pre-assessment Test

Exercises	Time/number of reps
Max rep push-up (Choose whichever variation of push-up you can execute with proper form)	☐
Notes: Record what you noticed. _____	
Squats for time (1 min)	☐
Notes: Record what you noticed. _____	
Plank hold for time (On hands or forearms)	☐
Notes: Record what you noticed. _____	

1 mile
(Run if you can; speed walk if you're not yet able)

Notes: Record what you noticed. _____

_____

Post-assessment Test

Exercises	Time/number of reps

Max rep push-up
(Choose whichever variation of push-up
you can execute with proper form)

Notes: Record what you noticed. _____

_____

Squats for time
(1 min)

Notes: Record what you noticed. _____

_____

Plank hold for time
(On hands or forearms)

Notes: Record what you noticed. _____

_____

1 mile
(Run if you can; speed walk if you're not yet able)

Notes: Record what you noticed. _____

_____

Max rep push-up: How many continuous push-ups did you do? Were they elevated? From your knees? When did you start to feel fatigued?

Squats for time: How many squats did you complete in one minute? Did you incorporate a load? If so, how much weight? When did you start to feel fatigued? Did you rest?

Plank hold for time: How long did you hold your plank? Were you balanced on your forearms? Your hands? When did you start to feel fatigued?

1 mile: Did you run or walk? When did you start to feel fatigued? Did you complete the mile without stopping to rest?

For more assessment tools, including ones for calculating your One-Rep Max (the max weight you can lift for a single repetition for a given exercise) or VO_2 Max (the maximum amount of oxygen you can utilize while working out), check out www.foreverstrongbook.com to download a template.

RESTING HEART RATE

Taking care of your heart and lungs can make a big difference for your quality of life, whether you're running to catch a train, a toddler, or a basketball at half-court. Who wants to get winded before they reach their target? To measure your resting heart rate, you can use a fitness watch, a heart-rate monitor, or just two fingers and the stopwatch feature on your phone. To manually determine your sixty-second heart rate in beats per minute (bpm):

1. Find your pulse over your radial artery (located on the thumb side of your wrist between the bone and the tendon).
2. Count the number of beats in fifteen seconds.
3. Multiply this number by four.

Did you land somewhere between 60 and 100 bpm? That's the range considered normal by the Mayo Clinic.[27] However, a lower resting heart rate corresponds with more efficient heart function, which implies better cardiovascular fitness. A highly trained athlete, for example, might normally have a rate of 40 bpm at rest.

Other factors that can influence a resting heart rate include:

- Age
- Activity
- Smoking status
- Cardiovascular disease, high cholesterol, or diabetes
- Body position (standing up or lying down, for example)
- Emotions
- Body size

Remember that becoming the person you wish to be requires taking action. Think of this physical reboot as a personal and mental reset as well. There is always room in life to gain new skills. Change does not demand perfect execution, but becoming the person you wish to be requires working through the journey. All along the way, you'll acquire traits that move you toward reaching your ultimate potential.

Embrace the challenge. Push yourself. That's the only way to know just how much your body can do. I'm thrilled to help show you what you're made of. Your body and mind are designed for resilience and strength. Exercise is your birthright. You are never too young or too old to start feeling amazing!

If you are a provider looking to incorporate Muscle-Centric Medicine® into your practice, go to www.drgabriellyon.com to sign up for my physicians' course to learn the foundations of nutrition, exercise, and the latest scientific research!

MINDSET RESET

OVERCOMING RESISTANCE

You can do hard things. The best version of yourself comes from cultivation, not comfort.

Human beings are complicated creatures. Influenced by thoughts and feelings that can override biological processes, people often respond to internal stimuli by making choices that can harm them over the long term. As we untangle the many intertwining aspects of health and wellness, we need to recognize all the complexities of human nature and account for *all* the inputs involved in obesity and other metabolic disorders.

Humans are also predictable. Our habits are consistent, and so is the language of resistance. I'm still amazed to discover, over and over, just how many different people get caught up in the same negative self-talk that seems hell-bent on keeping you small, holding you back from your goals, and distracting you from creating the life you want. My thought loops told me I would never be fit enough, which drove me to train for hours a day while neglecting other aspects of my life. It also kept me distracted by different exercise programs and allowed me to become reckless with my own well-being.

Remember, **YOU CANNOT NEGOTIATE with the voice of resistance**; it will talk you out of your dreams and the health you deserve. It will keep you in mediocre health, or worse. Do you take it personally when the thyroid produces thyroid hormone? Of course not. So don't take it personally when the brain produces thoughts, many of which are just noise that we need to learn to tune out. We cannot let defeatist thoughts rule.

Through practice, you can create a mental framework that accepts discomfort and maybe even embraces it as a sign of progress. You know that old saying that pain is just weakness leaving your body? Making change means growing, and growing isn't always comfortable. For example, we often interpret hunger as an emergency, even when it's not. This simple shift in reinterpreting your internal/physiological/physical cues can allow you to regain control.

With the Lyon Protocol, however, you won't often feel hungry, due to the power of amino acids. You might experience some hunger once you reach your physical goals and decide to blow past them and push even further. But when you do, remember it is a positive! While properly balancing micronutrients can go a long way toward minimizing hunger, the sensation itself, when it arises, can be reinterpreted as evidence that your body is utilizing stored fuel for energy. I typically tell my patients that hunger (not starvation) is something you can master. It is a cue that you are burning the excess adipose tissue keeping you from moving in the right direction.

Similarly, when it comes to exercise, I tell my patients, "If you don't want to quit at least once, you're not working hard enough." Hard is good. Human minds and bodies thrive under challenge, despite our tendency to seek out ways to make things easier.

We all struggle with resistance, which comes in many forms. You're tired and don't want to train. You had a stressful day, and the cookies are calling. You tell yourself all the different ways you are going to work out later, how it's counterproductive to train this late in the day, how more carbs will give you more energy. Time and time again, I have seen patients run through these same narratives in all different flavors. They sound like this:

- Food is my only joy in life. I cannot live without [*insert favorite food that keeps you further from your health goals*].
- I could never give up _____; it would make me sad.
- That takes too much work.
- Soothing myself with food is how I deal with my stress.
- I feel uncomfortable when I go out with my friends if I don't partake in what they're eating/drinking.
- It's not realistic to think I could just give up [*fill in the blank*].
- This is never going to work. I have tried everything.

Stop letting old habits hold you hostage!

The four most common excuses I hear that prevent people from reaching their wellness dreams are:

1. I don't have time.
2. No one really cares if I stay [overweight/in suboptimal health].
3. It probably won't work, so what is the point in trying?
4. The plan must be "realistic."

Here are some of my most common responses:

1. If you don't have time for fitness, how do you think you're going to have time for sickness? You're not ever going to

find the time for health; you must *make* the time. Think you're too busy to hit the gym? What does the log of your screen time have to say about that?

2. The way to make this process incredibly easy is to commit, 100 percent. You gain far more than muscle and lose more than fat when you dedicate yourself to achieving your goals.

3. Discard the things that matter least to make room for what matters most.

4. You are committing to and executing your plan not based on what others think but because your health is your responsibility.

5. The time is now. You will never get back this chance to become the best version of yourself. The sting of regret is real. Why look back on the goals you *could* have achieved?

We can always find excuses. Excuses won't get us where we want to be. We need to hold ourselves accountable.

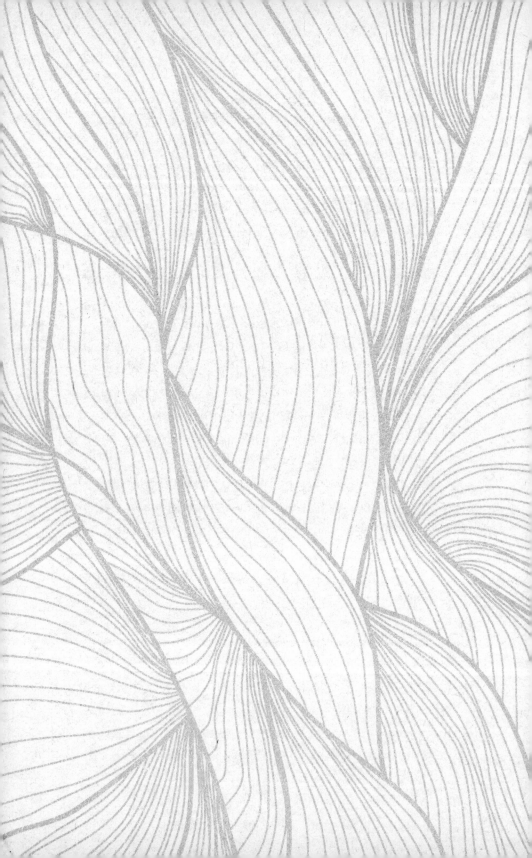

9.

~~~~~~~~

Training: The Minimum Effective Dose to Achieve the Maximum Result

E xercise is your body's birthright. We humans were designed for physical movement, and our bodies are capable of extraordinary feats. Don't think of training as an activity with health benefits. Instead, consider it as a baseline requirement for wellness and an essential component of maintaining health and protecting longevity.

Superior locomotion was essential for survival through much of human history. Back in the saber-toothed-tiger days, outmaneuvering both predators and prey depended upon physical prowess. Now the only hunting most of us do is for the charging cable when our phone battery dips to 1 percent. The only fleeing we do—at least, any of us who aren't pursued by paparazzi—is dodging someone we'd rather not talk to in the supermarket or at an office party.

Under the pressures of modern society, we can easily lose sight of the core physicality of our existence. Superficial vanity can strip away recognition of the beauty found in action—in challenging our bodies to power through difficult tasks and move in demanding ways. By pursuing fitness as an aesthetic, many of us have lost sight of exercising muscle as a vital element of basic daily living.

As we discussed in chapter 2, exercise is a first-line therapy to treat a wide array of diseases. You have the right to be healthy. You don't deserve to be in pain or to suffer. Isn't it empowering to know that you are entitled to be able to complete your daily tasks with ease—that you have the right to build the body armor (skeletal muscle) that will help protect you for the rest of your life? The Lyon Protocol prioritizes muscle as medicine, and training is a mandatory component. A well-designed program is essential. (*Pro tip:* Sitting on the couch and eating protein will not stimulate the muscle-protein synthesis your body needs!)

My workout programs prioritize not performance or looks (although both will, of course, get a nice boost along the way!) but disease prevention, treatment, and overall good health. Understanding muscle as the organ of longevity helps tune out the noise and minimize information overload. Instead of trying to incorporate every new tip or hack that pops up in your feed, try focusing strictly on building and protecting muscle. This approach will deliver big, long-lasting results in overall health and quality of life.

To become the architect of your own anatomy, first embrace the reality that movement is as important as brushing your teeth. We can all attest to the aches and pains in our backs and hips after sitting in a car, a plane, or a train or at a desk for hours on end. That's our body's way of saying, "Hey, you! I need to move! I wasn't designed to sit still!"

Training is nonnegotiable, because each passing "couch potato" year makes it harder and harder to get up and reverse course. You can expect to lose roughly 12 percent of your strength with each week of inactivity.[1] During periods of catabolic state (muscle loss or wasting) due to infection or injury, this loss can be even greater. Unfortunately, unforeseen periods of disuse inevitably occur. Whether you've discovered you're moving toward the deep end or just noticed you've been treading water for a while, this is the time to make a difference in your life.

EMPTY THE TANK (FAT ACCUMULATION IN MUSCLE)

We've already discussed how fat can accumulate in and around muscle, making the tissue look like a marbled steak. You now know that this lipid accumulation has been associated with accelerated aging, insulin resistance, diabetes, dyslipidemia, and obesity, as well as being a telltale sign of diabetes. An excess of intramuscular lipids leads to the buildup that inhibits insulin sensitivity and signaling. For this reason alone, there is no such thing as "healthy sedentary." Without exercise, muscle glycogen overfills muscle tissue, spilling out like an overpacked suitcase.

Testosterone, growth hormone, insulin, and essential amino acids all directly promote anabolism, meaning they contribute to building skeletal muscle and priming the body for growth. Exercise, meanwhile, further stimulates these growth effects. As we age, the natural production of testosterone and growth hormone declines, leaving lifestyle—primarily exercise—as the only natural way to increase and maintain previous levels. Meanwhile, low protein intake, cortisol spikes, illnesses, and stress carry catabolic effects. The more muscle tissue you have, the larger your reserves to defend against these challenges.

Resistance training plays a critical role here, increasing the potential for muscle-protein synthesis by amplifying the anabolic response to your pool of amino acids. In other words, the amino acids are like the gas in the tank, used during muscle contraction to build new muscle tissue. This is why eating the right amino acids is vital to your body's ability to maintain and build healthy muscle mass.

The rate of muscle-protein synthesis comes down to a ratio of muscle wasting versus muscle building. Our goal is to keep you on the positive side of rebuilding for as long as possible. This ebb-and-flow process is constant. As we age or become injured, our balance shifts from building to breakdown. It's not a question of *if* this will happen but *when*. In the meantime, we can build a body armor of muscle to prepare. You cannot wait to summon up the motivation to act. Your time is now.

To make this work, you need to want this change for yourself and to believe you have what it takes to achieve it. I'm arming you here with the information and tools you need to stop any cycle of excuses and stand up on your feet. By the end of this chapter, you'll know exactly how to get the results you seek.

REMODEL FOR MUSCLE

Exercise is traditionally divided into either endurance (cardio) or strength (weights). This is a fine starting point for understanding the different ends of the spectrum, but the interplay of different activity types is more complex, and many common beliefs around effective training haven't kept pace with research advancements. These days, lots of people lack knowledge, confidence, or both about how to integrate the types of exercise necessary to create proper training protocols. Too many remain confused about what, when, how, and why to work out.

> **Resistance exercise training** (RET) differs from endurance training, for example, and the specific challenges and benefits of each can help determine proper application. The goal of RET is to increase muscle mass and strength through regular high-tension muscle contractions against a heavy external load. Because of the muscle breakdown-and-repair process, training at least three times a week is essential. Performed regularly with enough load, this training generates the sequence of muscle breakdown and repair,

or hypertrophy, that builds new, stronger muscle tissue. The goal is providing a stimulus to drive adaptation.

Endurance exercise, on the other hand, involves long durations of low-tension muscle contractions that increase respiration, cardiac output, and blood flow. The resulting greater oxidative capacity improves cardiovascular function and fatigue resistance.[2]

High-intensity interval training (HIIT) is interval training exercise that calls for short bursts of activity followed by short periods of lower-intensity movements. HIIT incorporates several alternating rounds between several minutes of high-intensity movements—which increase the heart rate to at least 80 percent of your maximum heart rate—and periods of recovery during rest or less-demanding exercises. Because the training is framed around elevating your heart rate within a short period of time, HIIT can defend against the excuse "I don't have time to work out." Two popular versions of HIIT are Tabata and circuit training. The idea behind the HIIT approach is to gain results in a shorter amount of time, usually during thirty- to forty-five-minute sessions, or sometimes, as in the four-minute Tabata workout, even less.

Lots of workout confusion stems from the variations in training-program design. Building an individualized program involves multiple detailed considerations, and not everyone has the time or energy to invest in learning how to build a strong plan from scratch. Turning to a personal trainer can be a great solution, but not all trainers are created equal. The curriculum and continuing education requirements for different certifications vary tremendously.

The question then becomes, **how do I find a professional who can help me reach my goals?** Here are some insider tips:

- Before hiring a personal trainer, check for one of these well-respected accreditations: ACSM, NASM, ISSA, or NCSF, all of which come from certification programs that also offer internship and job-placement opportunities for graduates.
- Be sure that the trainer has experience working toward the specific goals you want to achieve. If you aim to build endurance for trail hiking or running cross-country, you may not want to pair with a trainer who only works with bodybuilders, for example.
- Check in on your progress after eight weeks. If you've done your part to keep your diet, sleep, and recovery on track for two months but see no noticeable progress, it's time to regroup. Discuss with your trainer how to achieve greater results. If you're still not convinced, it's time to find someone who is better suited for your individual needs.

I highly respect skilled trainers' abilities to help people transform their body composition, but I also want to empower *you* to understand how to get results in optimizing your muscle health. Let's dig into some of the science behind standard training recommendations and discuss how to design an exercise program, overcome common barriers, and understand the "why" behind it all.

There is one slam-dunk way to exercise wrong: don't do it at all.

First, it's important to understand your body type, fitness level, lifestyle, goals, and motivation for achieving them. Instead of being swayed by outside influences, base your personal standards on your individual needs and priorities. This will help you avoid either overshooting or underestimating your abilities.

Weekly Training Targets
- 150 minutes/week of moderate-intensity to vigorous exercise.
- Resistance training three to four days a week.
- 1 HIIT session each week.

Keys to Success
- Choose exercises that meet your current fitness level.
- Incorporate compound movements that involve more than one muscle group at a time.
- Prioritize proper sleep and nutrition.
- Continuously track your workouts and progressions.

CARDIO TRAINING

The more physically active you are, the more successfully you will keep your blood pressure down and maintain better levels of cholesterol and blood sugar. Aside from cardiac health, aerobic exercise (aka cardiorespiratory training) yields important metabolic benefits. Specifically, cardio increases capillary density,[3] which boosts the health of mitochondria by bringing nutrients and oxygen to body tissues.[4] **Training at varying intensities increases maximal oxygen uptake (VO_2 max), which is the maximum amount of oxygen you can utilize during exercise.** Increasing your VO_2 max over time will allow you to sustain energy through longer periods of activity. And given that a reduced VO_2 max is the strongest predictor of cardiovascular and all-cause mortality (aka your likelihood of dying), it's an excellent measure for health.

HEART RATE

Calculating your heart rate during activity is an important gauge of training effort. A comprehensive training program includes target heart-rate ranges for different cardio-focused workouts. Remember how to calculate your sixty-second heart rate in bpm? Measure your fifteen-second pulse and multiply that number by four.

RESISTANCE TRAINING

Cardio is essential for good health, but the benefits expand exponentially once you add in resistance training. Not only will strength training create more muscle tissue to act as your metabolic sink (the ability to take up nutrients such as glucose and fatty acids), but combining cardio with resistance training on the regular will also keep you from gaining back any fat you've lost, eliminating the yo-yo effect of dieting.

Increasing strength-training output remains one of the most effective tools to move the body-composition needle—especially if you've been feeling stuck. Due to the rapid turnover of muscle tissue, consistent training is vital to your health. Simply put, resistance training breaks down muscles, and then protein yields repair. Protein builds muscle through muscle-protein synthesis, the process by which you grow stronger and gain muscle definition. As you know by now, developing healthy muscle tissue can determine your body composition for a lifetime.

The first adjustment I usually make to a patient's plan is upping their resistance training. Next, I often add HIIT, which involves intense bouts of exercise—pushing to at least 80 percent of maximal heart rate—interspersed with recovery periods of lower-intensity exercise or rest.

To guide you as you build your own plan, here are the benchmarks I recommend for those at beginner, intermediate, and advanced levels, as established by the ACSM.

BEGINNER (Baseline Level)
- At least 150 minutes of moderate-intensity aerobic training per week.
OR
- 75 minutes of vigorous aerobic physical activity.
OR
- an equivalent combination of moderate intensity and vigorous aerobic activity per week.
PLUS
- Resistance training of moderate or greater intensity that involves all major muscle groups at least two days a week.
OR
- Full-body resistance two days a week.

INTERMEDIATE
- At least 150 minutes of vigorous aerobic training per week.
- Resistance training of moderate or greater intensity that involves all major muscle groups three to four times a week, using eight to twelve reps per exercise.

ADVANCED
- At least 150 minutes of vigorous aerobic training per week.
- Resistance training of high intensity that involves all major muscle groups four to six times per week, adapted to your specific goals.

Determine Your Training Status

Training status	Training experience	Time of detraining (no training or exercise)	Exercise technique/form
Beginner	Up to 2 months	8 or more months	Developing
Intermediate	Between 2 and 12 months	Between 4 and 8 months	Good
Advanced	Between 1 and 3 years	Between 1 and 4 months	Excellent

I often hear of people concerned and frustrated about not seeing results either working with a trainer or on their own. Let's discuss a couple of reasons why that might be.

1 The lack of progressive overload. This means you are not gradually increasing the difficulty of your workout as your body is adapting to the current stress/demand of the exercises.

2 Lack of adherence. This means you're not actually sticking to your plan.

The solution is to create a plan that works within your parameters. Your exercise routine must work with your life—including job obligations, kids' schedules, or travel plans—not against it. Sure, I've mentioned the recommended frequency of training based on your status, but any plan that doesn't work with your nonnegotiable life commitments is only setting you up to fail. We want a program that will allow you to stay consistent and deliver results.

Step one is to identify your training goal. Goal setting is one of the most overlooked elements of programming. Skipping this aspect leaves you without clear direction about what you should be doing either at home or in the gym. Do you walk into your workouts with a program written down and ready to go? Or do you wander around the weight machines, wondering what to do until you end up choosing exercises at random? Do you get intimidated by all the gym equipment and wind up slinking back to the cardio section? Having a clear and specific training goal can help you push back against feeling overwhelmed.

It is critical to discover **where you are, where you want to go, and what is the optimal way to get there**. If you tend to skip over this step, you most likely have not achieved the results you desired. One way to identify a training goal and keep yourself on track is by creating a SMART goal (Specific, Measurable, Action-oriented, Realistic, and Timely).

5 TIPS FOR SETTING REALISTIC FITNESS GOALS

➡ Use visualization to find your "Why"

➡ Break big goals down into smaller parts

➡ Create daily goal-supporting habits

➡ Create challenging but achievable goals

➡ Enjoy the struggle

SMART GOAL EXAMPLE

Sex: Female

Age: 40

Current body-fat percentage: 35 percent

Training level: Intermediate

GOAL

Specific: I want to lose weight so I can hike a trail easily with my family.

Measurable: I want to drop 10 percent body fat.

Action-oriented: I am going to work out five days a week.

Realistic or relevant: Full-body resistance training and regular cardio will translate to my goal of hiking and is realistic with my schedule.

TIP

To ensure that your goal is realistic, consider these factors:

- How old are you?
- What is your training experience?
- How much time do you have to commit to your training?

Since we tend to get overzealous and sometimes shoot for the stars, one approach is to subtract 10 percent from the goal you originally created.

Timely: A weekly milestone would be to exercise five times a week, while a long-term goal would be to stick with this program for six months.

Final SMART goal: I want to lose 10 percent body fat so I can enjoy hiking with my family. To get me there, I am going to do three days of full-body resistance training at home and two days of cardiovascular training each week to prepare me for my hiking trip in six months.

Record your own SMART goal here:

_____

_____

_____

_____

After you have identified your one (or two, max) SMART goals, we need to identify any roadblocks that could impede your progress. Write down all your commitments and anything that might keep you from accomplishing your goal. What time do you have to be at work? What time do you have to pick up the kids or take them to a practice or event? What if they're home sick? Do you have a recurring injury? Do you travel frequently? Write down all the nonnegotiables and commitments you have in your schedule along with some potential solutions for when they arise.

Example: I start work at 8:30 a.m. every day. I travel once a month for business. I must complete all my independent activities by 8:00 p.m. to preserve quality time with my family.

→ If life gets in the way of a formal workout, I commit to doing 15 push-ups, 25 air squats, and a fast-paced walk around the neighborhood.

→ If I'm on a business trip, I will use the hotel gym or do a body-weight workout in my hotel room in the morning. My main priority while traveling will be to optimize my nutrition.

Write down your roadblocks and some alternatives for when issues arise:

_____

_____

_____

_____

Next, we're going to determine your goal timeline and your weekly training frequency. Look ahead on your calendar and see what you have planned. Based on your schedule, decide on a realistic timeline for reaching your goal—three months, six months, one year? Can you slot in training sessions five days each week? You can always add more days—just be sure to set a baseline target that you can hit every week.

Example: I will lose 10 percent body fat in six months through resistance training three days a week and cardio twice a week.

Record your own SMART goal timeline:

_____

_____

_____

Now that we've clarified your SMART goal(s), identified nonnegotiable commitments, anticipated potential obstacles to consistency, and framed your training frequency and timeline, let's move on to exercise selection.

FOUNDATIONS OF TRAINING

Different phases of training lead to specific physical adaptations. Choose each specific phase based on your training level as well as your SMART goal. Below are the five phases, according to the National Academy of Sports Medicine.[5]

1. **Stabilization:** The ability to provide dynamic joint support to maintain correct posture during all movements. This is a good starting point for beginners to build a foundation before adding additional load (or weights) to exercises.
2. **Muscular endurance:** The ability to produce and maintain force over prolonged periods.
3. **Muscular hypertrophy:** Increasing muscle size through enlargement of skeletal-muscle fibers.
4. **Muscular strength:** The neuromuscular system's ability to produce internal tension to overcome external force. (It's critical to establish solid stabilization before moving on to this adaptation.)
5. **Muscular power:** The neuromuscular system's ability to produce the greatest possible force in the shortest amount of time possible. Think explosive movements.

For the purposes of this book, we will focus on beginner and intermediate levels, pairing muscular endurance with cardiovascular training. For more adaptations aimed at different fitness levels, visit www.foreverstrongbook.com, where you'll find sample programs for a variety of training goals.

The Warm-up

Far too many people skip this essential aspect of training, which is arguably the most important for preventing injury. The warm-up prepares your body for the exercises in the coming workout by increasing your range of motion, improving blood flow to the muscles, and generally activating your system in advance of training intensity.

A dynamic warm-up that includes movement rather than static stretches can start with five minutes of cardiovascular activity (treadmill, StairMaster, high knees in place) at low to moderate intensity followed by five to fifteen minutes of more specific movements based on the day's exercises. Important areas to warm up are the ankle complex, the hip complex, and the thoracic spine in your mid-back. A warm-up is essential on your cardio days as well.

Exercise Selection and Rules of Engagement

Here are tips for choosing which exercises to include in your program.

- Select exercises you know how to properly execute. Correct form is the foremost priority with *any* exercise.
- Create a balance between muscle groups and movement patterns. Train each specific muscle group three to five times per week with 48 to 72 hours of recovery time in between.
- Think of ways you can make your current exercise selection more challenging once you're ready to progress. Adding more load (weight)? Increasing time under tension?
- Your performance will reflect the quality of your sleep and nutrition. Keep recovery as a high priority, or your training will suffer.
- *Bonus tip:* For a higher payoff, do your conditioning and interval work as a separate morning session, then complete a resistance training session approximately six to eight hours later. Research suggests that back-to-back strength and endurance sessions are less effective because of insufficient recovery time to achieve maximal benefit.[6] But this type of scheduling is an

ideal, not a requirement. Most important is that you get the sessions done.

At this point, you may be feeling a little overwhelmed by all this information. Take time to absorb it. Then settle in as I offer you a framework that can help simplify how to get started. There is no one way to design programs, but my goal is to arm you with the basics to build confidence around exercising.

Remember that your body is three-dimensional. This may sound obvious, but too often I see people working out who seem to have forgotten that their bodies can move in ways other than forward and backward (referred to as the sagittal plane of movement). Our bodies also have the capacity to move laterally (side to side) and to rotate. A well-rounded program requires balance between muscle groups and incorporates all our movement patterns. Your workout also needs to balance pulling motions (e.g., a row, bicep curl, lat pull-down) with pushing motions (e.g., push-up, chest press, overhead press). Leg exercises occupy their own category, beyond push or pull, because most incorporate both the anterior (front) and posterior (back) muscles synergistically, unless specific muscles are isolated on a machine.

Balancing your workouts among the push, pull, and leg categories can help reduce feeling overwhelmed by deciding which combinations of exercise to choose. Next, it's time to tie in planes of motion. For example, a chest press is like an overhead press in terms of mechanics, but the movement takes place in a different plane of motion. The muscle groups targeted in each of those exercises are different due to the positioning of the weights in space.

Tip: Perform the most important exercises first, when you have the most energy, mental focus, and time. Prioritizing which movements you execute at your peak will bring you that much closer to achieving your goal. If your workout winds up getting cut short, at least you will have consistently executed your workout's primary objective.

MIND-MUSCLE CONNECTION

Exercise starts in the brain. You can use physical training not only to jack up your strength but also to sharpen your attention skills. Several studies show that muscle improvement increases when we visualize the target muscle and consciously direct activity and concentration there during exercise performance. For example, in a bicep curl, focus your attention on the squeeze in the bicep at the top of every rep. Every exercise requires a mind-muscle connection.

Your intention is key. Directed attention correlates with increased activation, possibly reducing contribution from other muscles. Before you begin your workout, silence your phone and get your mind in the zone. Ignoring the ping of texts and alerts will help you focus on the muscle you're targeting in each exercise. Over the long term, this approach can improve your training, both mentally and physically.[7]

And now . . . here's a dumbbell-only program focused on muscular endurance and cardiovascular training that's geared toward those at a beginner/intermediate training level. (For more advanced training program options, check out www.foreverstrongbook.com.)

This program is designed to be accessible to everyone, whether at home or in the gym.

Let's take another look at our previous example.

SMART goal: I want to lose 10 percent body fat so I can enjoy hiking with my family. To get me there, I am going to do three days a week of full-body resistance training at home and two days of cardiovascular training to prepare me for my hiking trip in six months.

Nonnegotiables and commitments that could get in the way of your goal: I start work at 8:30 a.m. every day, I travel once a month for business, and I must stop independent activities by 8:00 p.m. to protect quality time with my family. I will plan to do my workouts at home in the morning.

Time frame and training frequency: Three days of resistance training and two days of cardio.

Monday: Resistance training, full body
Tuesday: Low-impact cardio
Wednesday: Resistance training, full body
Thursday: High-impact cardio
Friday: Resistance training, full body

WORKOUT INSTRUCTIONS

Equipment needed: dumbbells (learn more about starting-weight selection on page 263), bench (optional)

Block A: Warm-up (body-weight exercises)
Block B: First circuit (dumbbells)
Block C: Second circuit (dumbbells)
Cooldown: Downregulated breathing such as box breathing: inhale for four seconds, hold for four seconds, exhale for four seconds, hold for four seconds, and repeat.

1. Complete two rounds of block A (the warm-up) with zero seconds of rest between rounds.

2. Then move on to block B exercises and complete as many rounds as possible (AMRAP) within those ten minutes.

3. Take a two-minute rest.

4. Then perform ten minutes of block C exercises AMRAP.

5. Cooldown. Done.

Additional Notes

■ For all unilateral (one-sided) movements, perform the programmed number of reps on each side.

■ In the Reps column below, you will see an e for unilateral movement. The e stands for "each side." DB = dumbbell. Alt. = alternate the left and right sides.

■ Before you begin, please refer to www.foreverstrongbook.com to review the video library of exercises.

■ See page 263 for information on how to select your starting weight for each exercise.

FIVE-DAY TRAINING PROGRAM

DAY 1—FULL BODY

Exercises	Rounds	Reps	Rest
A1 **Squat to reach**	2	5	
Notes: _____			
A2 **Hip flexor stretch**		20 sec e	0
Notes: _____			
10 min AMRAP			
B1 **Alt. DB chest press**		15 e	
Notes: _____			

B2	DB underhand grip row	15	

Notes: _____

B3	DB split squat	15 e	0

Notes: _____

Rest 2 minutes, then move on to next AMRAP

10 min AMRAP

C1	Reverse crunch	10	

Notes: _____

C2	Side plank elbow to knee	10 e	

Notes: _____

C3	Bear crawls	10 e	Done

Notes: _____

DAY 1 EXERCISE LIBRARY

WARM-UP BLOCK A

Squat to reach. This warms up the hips and allows extension and rotation of the thoracic spine. Take your time, and focus on breathing throughout the exercise.

1. Start with your feet in a wide stance, with your feet slightly past your shoulders in a sumo-squat stance.
2. Drop into a deep squat (as low as you can go).
3. Place your right elbow against your knee, and push your knee out slightly with your elbow as your left arm reaches toward the ceiling. Let your eyes follow your left hand.
4. Then move to the other side, placing your left elbow against your left knee and pushing your knee out with your elbow as your

body twists and your right arm reaches up toward the ceiling. Your eyes will follow your right hand.

5. Come back to center in the squat position. Reach both arms up in a V position over your head, and stand up from the squat.

6. Repeat for 5 repetitions.

Hip flexor stretch. This warms up the hip flexor.

1. Assume a half-kneeling position with your left knee on the floor and your right foot forward.

2. Squeeze your glutes (your butt) to engage your left quad up past your hip flexor.

3. In this position, take some deep breaths, and you'll start to feel your hip flexors opening up after each deep breath.

4. Hold for 20 seconds, and switch to the other side.

5. Go back to the squat to reach, and complete another round of the warm-up.

AMRAP BLOCK B

Alternating DB chest press. The purpose of doing alternating chest press is to increase the time your muscle is under tension, which will increase your heart rate and make it more challenging while working the chest, shoulders, and triceps. This exercise is also great for your core, which must stay engaged to stabilize the movement.

1. This can be done on a bench or on the floor.

2. Start with both dumbbells (weight of your choice) at the top, keeping both dumbbells in line with your shoulders.

3. Lower your right dumbbell into the chest press position while stabilizing with your raised left arm continuing to hold the left dumbbell up in the air.

4. Push the right arm back to the starting position, and then lower the left arm while stabilizing the right side with the right dumbbell kept raised.

5. Perform 15 repetitions on each arm for a total of 30 repetitions.

DB underhand grip row. This exercise is going to work your lats (back) and biceps.

1. Stand with your feet about shoulder-width apart, holding a dumbbell in each hand.

2. Turn your palms so they are facing forward, and lean your upper body forward about 45–90 degrees while keeping your back as flat as possible.

3. Pull your elbows back while squeezing the shoulder blades together. You want to think of your hands reaching back toward your pants pockets as your elbows drive back.

4. Straighten your arms back down to the starting position.

5. Complete 15 repetitions.

DB split squat. This exercise will work your quads, hamstrings, glutes, and hip complex.

1. Start with a dumbbell in each hand, and move your feet into a staggered stance with one foot forward and the other foot back, standing on the ball of your back foot with your heel raised.

2. Lower into the squat position, maintaining a 90-degree angle in the front leg. (Don't let your knee move forward over your toes.) Keep your upper body vertical throughout the exercise.

3. Press back up to the starting position.

4. Complete 15 repetitions on each leg.

5. Start back at the top of the circuit with the alt. DB chest press, and keep going until your 10-minute timer rings.

AMRAP BLOCK C

Reverse crunch. This exercise is a core scorcher. Get ready for the burn in your abs.

1. This exercise can be done on the floor or a bench.
2. Lie on your back, and bring your feet up to the ceiling, keeping a slight bend in the knees. If you feel too much tension in your lower back in this position, make a triangle with your hands, and place them under your tailbone.
3. Lower your feet to the floor. The goal is to lower your feet to just two inches above the floor, but start with what's achievable for you now, and work your way toward lowering your legs farther while keeping your lower back flat.

Side plank with elbow to knee. This exercise works your obliques.

1. Lie on your side with your elbow under your shoulder. You can stack your feet on top of each other or have them in a staggered position where one foot is in front of the other.
2. Push your hips up toward the ceiling to assume the side plank position, keeping the top edge of your body in an even straight line.
3. Reach your top arm above your head, and lift your top foot away from the foot that's on the ground. Bend your elbow and knee so they touch, and then extend back out to the starting position.
4. Complete 10 repetitions, and repeat on the other side.

Note: If the elbow to knee is too challenging for you, start by lying on your side with your elbow on the floor in line with your shoulder. Bend your knees so your feet are behind you, with your knees in a line with your hips. You should be in one flat line with your feet behind you. Push your hips up to the ceiling, hold, and then lower. Repeat 10 times, and then switch to the other side.

Bear crawls. This engages the entire body and increases heart rate.

1. Start on all fours with your toes tucked.
2. Lift your knees off the ground.
3. Crawl forward by moving your left knee toward your left elbow and simultaneously moving your right arm forward. Now move your right knee toward your right elbow, and simultaneously move your left arm forward. Continue crawling forward for 10 repetitions on each side or a total of 20. Try to keep your knees as close to the floor as possible to challenge the core. You can perform either 20 bear crawls forward or 10 forward and 10 backward.
4. Once this block is complete, start back with the first exercise, and keep going through the rounds until your 10-minute timer rings.

DAY 2—LOW-IMPACT CARDIO

Note: Don't forget to warm up on your cardio days!

Choose your favorite form of low-impact cardio. Examples: swimming, biking, rowing, elliptical, hiking, walking.

Low-intensity exercise means working within 50 to 60 percent of your max heart rate. Any of the examples listed above will qualify. Or calculate it yourself with this equation: 220 − your age = general guideline for max heart rate. Then multiply that number times the percentage of the target heart-rate zone.

DAY 3—FULL BODY			
Exercises	**Rounds**	**Reps**	**Rest**
A1 **Squat prying**	2	20 sec	
Notes: _____			
A2 **T's, Y's, L's, W's**		8 e	0
Notes: _____			

10 min AMRAP

B1 **Kickstand RDL**		10 e	
Notes: _____			
B2 **Push-ups**		10	
Notes: _____			
B3 **DB bridge pullover**		10	0
Notes: _____			

Rest 2 minutes, then move on to next AMRAP

10 min AMRAP

C1 **Goblet squat**		15	
Notes: _____			
C2 **DB curls**		15	
Notes: _____			
C3 **DB kickbacks**		15	Done
Notes: _____			

DAY 3 EXERCISE LIBRARY

WARM-UP BLOCK A

Squat prying. This warms up the hip complex and the spine.

1. Start in a wide-stance squat with your toes pointed slightly out.
2. Squat down as low as you can, and place both elbows against the inside of the knees.
3. Press your elbows out to drive your knees open, and lift your chest. Take some deep breaths, and hold for 20 seconds.

T's, Y's, L's, W's. These warm up your shoulder complex and back. (You can add 5-pound dumbbells to these exercises if you'd like.)

1. **T's.** Bend your upper body forward 45–90 degrees with your knees slightly bent.
2. Put your arms straight in front of you (your arms should be in line with your chest), and rotate your palms forward.
3. Bring your arms straight to your sides, and bring them back to the starting position. Move at a quick pace, swinging to the side and back down, making a T shape.
4. Complete 8 repetitions.
5. **Y's.** Assume the previous position, but this time, instead of your arms making a T, they are going to make a Y.
6. Starting in the same bent-over position with your arms in front of you, in line with your chest, turn your palms to face each other, and swing your arms out to a Y so your arms are in line with your head.
7. Complete 8 repetitions.
8. **L's.** Starting in the same bent-over position, bring your elbows back to create a 90-degree angle like you would make in a push-up position.
9. From here, keep the elbows where they are, and flip your hands up like you're under arrest. Reverse it, and come back to the starting position.
10. Complete 8 repetitions.

11. **W's.** Staying in the same bent-over position, make a 90-degree angle with your palms facing you (it will almost look like a bicep curl).

12. From here, keep the 90-degree angle, swing your arms to your sides, squeeze your back at the top, and swing back down, making a W shape.

13. Complete 8 repetitions, and then return to squat prying, completing one more round of the warm-up.

AMRAP BLOCK B

Kickstand RDL. This works the hamstrings.

1. Holding a dumbbell in each hand, assume a staggered-stance position with one foot forward and one foot back, with the toes tucked and heels off the floor (acting as a kickstand).

2. From here, shift your body forward to transfer 90 percent of your weight over your front leg.

3. Visualize wearing a knee and back brace so that the only way you can move forward is by pushing your butt and hips back. Bend at the hips to complete the dead-lift motion.

4. Keep the two dumbbells directly in line with your front leg, imagining that you're pressing the weights against your front leg the whole time. Keeping the dumbbells close will prevent you from straining your lower back.

5. Next, push your hips forward to bring your upper body back to the starting position.

6. Complete 10 repetitions, and switch to the other side.

Push-ups. This is a full-body exercise.

1. Start in a plank position, squeeze your glutes, engage your back, and complete 10 repetitions of the push-up. Perform a standard

push-up if you're able. Other options include placing your knees on the floor or elevating your hands on a platform.

DB bridge pullover. This works the glutes, hamstrings, and lats—especially helpful if you spend much of your day sitting.

1. Start with one lighter dumbbell.
2. Lie on your back, place your feet on the floor, and hold the dumbbell with both hands.
3. From here, push the hips up toward the ceiling while pushing the dumbbell up toward the ceiling.
4. Keeping your arms straight, lower the dumbbell back toward the floor in line with your head, and drive it back toward the starting position. *Note:* Your hips will remain off the floor in the glute bridge position the entire time.
5. Complete 10 repetitions. Return to the first exercise, and keep going through the round until your 10-minute timer goes off.

AMRAP BLOCK C

Goblet squat. This works the lower body and core.

1. Stand with your feet about shoulder-width apart.
2. Holding one dumbbell in two hands, brace it against your chest.
3. Bend down into the squat, and drive back up, keeping the weight in the same position by the chest.
4. Complete 15 repetitions.

DB curls. This works the biceps.

1. Start in a narrow stance with your feet about hip-distance apart, holding a dumbbell in each hand.
2. Starting with your arms by your sides and palms facing forward, curl the dumbbells up, and control them on the way down.

Think of keeping your elbows in one position so that the only thing moving is your hands curling up and down.

3. Complete 15 repetitions.

DB kickbacks. These work the triceps.

1. Start with a dumbbell in each hand. Bend forward, squeezing your back muscles to keep them engaged, and send your elbows back.

2. Holding this position, extend your arms behind you (feeling a contraction in the triceps), and then return them to the bent-elbow position.

3. The key is to not move the arms up and down. Hold still except for extending the arm behind you. Keep your back as flat as possible.

4. Complete 15 repetitions, and then return to the first exercise. Keep completing the round until your 10-minute timer rings.

DAY 4—HIGH-IMPACT CARDIO

Note: Don't forget to warm up on your cardio days!

Choose your favorite form of high-impact cardio. Examples: HIIT class, sprint intervals, running, StairMaster, boxing.

High-intensity cardio entails working at 70 to 80 percent of your max heart rate. Either choose one of the activities above or calculate your heart-rate range using this formula: 220 – your age = general guideline for max heart rate. Then multiply that number times the percentage of the target heart-rate zone.

DAY 5—FULL BODY

Exercises	Rounds	Reps	Rest
A1 **Thoracic bridge**	2	3 e	
Notes: _____			
A2 **Plank walkouts**		10	0
Notes: _____			

10 min AMRAP

B1 **Alt. lunges**		15 e	
Notes: _____			
B2 **Alt. DB shoulder press**		15 e	
Notes: _____			
B3 **DB reverse fly**		15	0
Notes: _____			

Rest 2 minutes, then move on to next AMRAP

10 min AMRAP

C1 **DB side raise**	10 min AMRAP	10	
Notes: _____			
C2 **Plank touches**		10 e	
Notes: _____			
C3 **Single-arm suitcase carry**		15 steps (e)	Done
Notes: _____			

DAY 5 EXERCISE LIBRARY

WARM-UP BLOCK A

Thoracic bridge. This warms up the hip and shoulder complex.

1. Start in a downward dog position.
2. Drop into the bear crawl position.
3. Lift one hand off the ground, and rotate outward so both feet are on the ground and the front of your body is facing the ceiling.
4. From here, push the hips up, and reach the hand that is off the floor back over your head.
5. Take some deep breaths, and return to the starting position, then rotate to the other side.
6. Complete 3 repetitions on each side.

Plank walkouts. These work on your hinge, hamstring, shoulders, and core.

1. Begin by standing upright, then reach down like you're going to touch your toes. (If needed, bend your knees to lessen the tension on the hamstrings.)
2. From here, walk out into a plank position.
3. Walk back toward your feet, and repeat 10 times.
4. Return to the thoracic bridge to complete another round of each exercise.

AMRAP BLOCK B

Alternating lunges. This is a lower-body exercise.

1. Start in a standing position. You can hold dumbbells or perform with body weight only.

2. Step one leg forward into a lunge, and push back to return to the starting position.

3. Repeat on the other leg to complete 15 repetitions on each side, or a total of 30 repetitions.

Alternating DB shoulder press. This works the shoulders, triceps, and core.

1. Start in a narrow stance with feet about hip-width apart.

2. Bring both dumbbells into position for the shoulder press (your arms to the sides of you with elbows facing outward).

3. From here, press the right arm up while stabilizing the left arm. Bring the right arm back down, and then press the left arm up.

Note: If shoulder mobility constraints mean you can't complete the exercise without leaning back, switch to a neutral position. Instead of your palms facing forward and your elbows out to your sides, bring the elbows in so your palms face each other.

4. Complete 15 repetitions on each side for a total of 30 repetitions.

DB reverse fly. This works the upper posterior chain (upper back). Go lighter for this exercise.

1. Start in a standing position, holding both dumbbells.

2. With your knees slightly bent, bend over, keeping your back flat, to a 45- to 90-degree angle.

3. Place your arms in front of you so your palms are facing each other, keeping your hands in line with your chest.

4. From here, fly your arms out to the sides, and squeeze your shoulder blades together at the top.

5. Return to the starting position, and complete 15 repetitions.

6. Return to the first exercise, and continue going through the round until your 10-minute timer rings.

AMRAP BLOCK C

DB side raise. This works the deltoid (outer area of the shoulder).

1. Start in a narrow stance with feet about hip-width apart, holding light- to moderate-weight dumbbells.
2. Bend the elbows slightly, then raise the dumbbells to your sides until they reach shoulder height (don't go above the level of your shoulders). Return to the starting position.
3. Complete 10 repetitions.

Plank touches. This works your core.

1. Place an object on the floor at arm's length in front of you. (You can use a med ball, a dumbbell, your shoe, etc.) Assume a plank position with your feet in a wide stance.
2. Lift your left hand off the floor, and reach to touch the object. Return it to the floor, then repeat the movement with your right hand. Keep your hips locked in place without shifting your weight.
3. Complete a set of 10 repetitions on each arm for a total of 20 repetitions.

Single-arm suitcase carry. This is a core exercise.

1. Hold a dumbbell in one hand. The goal of this exercise is to engage your core so completely that the dumbbell cannot pull you over off your center. Squeeze the muscles in your core as a counterforce against where the weight is pulling you.
2. Walk forward, keeping your shoulders balanced.
3. Complete 15 steps holding the weight with the right hand, and then switch the dumbbell to the left hand and complete another 15 steps.

4. Return to the first exercise, and continue going through the round until your 10-minute timer rings.

Variables you can manipulate to progress the difficulty after four weeks:
- Repetitions
- Sets
- Training intensity
- Repetition tempo
- Training volume (or load)
- Rest intervals
- Training frequency
- Training duration
- Exercise selection

FAQS

Q. How do I select my starting weight?

A. Everyone starts at a different strength level. When selecting weights, I recommend starting easy during the first week. Get familiar with the program and track your weights. (Use the Notes spaces to track your weights as well as recording any observations.) The goal of my programming is to work up to one to two reps away from failure. In other words, when completing sets with a particular weight, you should have enough "gas left in the tank" to complete one or two more reps. Never sacrifice form to increase weight.

Q. What do I do when the number of rounds or reps increases from one week to the next?

A. You should try to maintain the same weight you used in the previous week.

Q. What do I do when the number of rounds or reps decreases from one week to the next?

A. You should try to increase the weight from what you used in the previous week.

Q. **What do I do when the number of reps remains the same from one week to the next?**

A. You should try to increase the weight from what you used in the previous week.

Q. **How do I know when it's time to increase the weight on a particular exercise?**

A. If you complete your last set and still have enough strength to complete an additional three to five reps, then it is time to increase the weight. Don't be afraid to go heavy, as long as you don't sacrifice form.

Q. **How can I increase the weight when heavier equipment isn't available?**

A. Resistance bands, a weighted vest, adding time under tension (TUT), and decreasing the rest time between sets are all great options.

Q. **What should I do when a unilateral exercise is programmed?**

A. For all unilateral (one-sided) movements, perform the programmed number of reps on each side. In the Reps column, you will see an e for unilateral movement. The e stands for "each side." Exercises labeled alternating (alt.), single-arm, or single-leg are easy to identify as unilateral movements. However, there are other unilateral movements that don't have these indicator words, such as walking lunges, hip flexor stretches, side planks, bear crawls, and so on.

Q. **What should I do when one side is weaker than the other?**

A. This is a common issue. Begin with your weaker side. Keep track of the weights. This will even out over time. Make sure that you are executing the reps with proper form. Quality over quantity.

Q. Why is there no rest time programmed during the A block?

A. I never program rest during the warm-up (A block). The warm-up is meant to increase your heart rate and therefore your blood flow, which enables more oxygen to reach your muscles. The movements are not overly strenuous, and you should not need to rest between the rounds. However, if you need rest, take it!

Q. What are some other cooldown options?

A. Select an activity that will gradually reduce your heart rate. Gently stretching each of the main muscle groups will bring both your body and your mind back to a resting state, or do the breathing exercises mentioned under "Workout Instructions" above.

Q. How do I know if I am completing the exercises properly?

A. You can find a video tutorial for each exercise at www.foreverstrong book.com.

Q. What's the difference between pain and soreness?

A. Pain means you need to avoid the movement and see a doctor. Soreness, on the other hand, is an expected part of starting a new program. Struggling to differentiate? Pain, typically characterized as sharp and persistent, develops quickly and lasts longer than a couple of days even without any movement. Soreness, which is temporary, comes on slowly and can feel like muscle burning or tightness. One type of soreness, lasting from 24 to 48 hours, is called delayed-onset muscle soreness (DOMS) and can occur after intense and heavy-weight workouts. To aid your post-workout recovery, make sure to stretch, rest, and eat high-quality foods.

Q. How can I track my progress?

A. I am old-school. I like to track my progress in a handwritten journal. The Notes spaces in the program are meant for you to track
your weights and observations. I suggest you find a way that works
best for you and stick to that format. Consistency is important.

Q. What is an NSV?

A. Nonscale victory! These are improvements that may go unnoticed
if you are only focused on the scale. Examples include your clothes
fitting better, feeling more active with your family, having more
energy for life, improved sleep, losing inches not pounds, improved
mental health, and improved medical markers (blood pressure and
blood-sugar levels). Your health journey is so much more than a
number on a scale.

Q. How do I record a starting point before the program?

A. Take pictures! You don't have to post them anywhere. While you
are burning fat, you are also gaining muscle. The scale will not tell
the whole story. Before-and-after photos are a great way to track
body composition changes.

Q. I am not seeing results. What now?

A. Take an honest look at your day. What are you doing with the
other twenty-three hours? Training for one hour per day and then
spending the remainder of the day anchored to a desk or motion-
less on the sofa will not lead to massive results. In addition to this
program, I highly recommend taking around 10,000 steps per day.
If you are nowhere near 10,000, just focus on improving.

Q. Which is more important, consistency or intensity?

A. Consistency. Once consistency is mastered, you can start focusing on your intensity.

There you have it! We've reviewed the science of why you should exercise, discussed how to implement a program that works with your life, covered the basics of program design, and explored why you may not have seen results in the past. Remember, it's never too late to get started. Create small, tangible goals, stay consistent, and experience the life you deserve!

POWER HACKS

- **You can't out-train a bad diet.**
- **Complete your workout at least six hours away from bedtime.** If this is not possible with your schedule, that's OK, if it's not negatively affecting your sleep.
- **Complete your hardest workouts on the days you typically feel more rested and have the most energy.**
- **Execute the most important exercise in your program first.** If a roadblock cuts your workout short, you'll still have accomplished the most important elements to drive you toward your goal.
- **Recovery matters too.** Check in with yourself about your relationship with exercise. If your body is craving rest yet you feel anxiety about missing one workout, explore possible root causes of that emotion. Work on reframing your perspective so exercise is an asset, not something that controls your life.

Check out www.foreverstrongbook.com for my program templates for hypertrophy, maximal strength, power, and more!

MINDSET RESET

FIVE FUNDAMENTAL ATTRIBUTES

Let's think of our work together as constructing the house of your dreams. The building blocks consist of the five fundamental attributes that each of us has within. These are:

1. **Courage**
2. **Perseverance**
3. **Self-discipline**
4. **Adaptability**
5. **Resilience**

All of us have some hardwiring to contend with if we want to make change. The filter through which you process information and experiences is determined by the combination of your inborn attributes and the inner dialogue/self-talk that strengthens or diminishes them. Each attribute is a superpower that, with practice, can be maximized to help bridge the gap between who you are today (your current self) and who you want to become (your future self).

Many of us have grown accustomed to routinely analyzing these traits in the context of our careers, but rarely do we examine their role in creating and executing a wellness plan. Underdeveloped fundamental attributes are one reason you may have struggled in the past to follow a plan and achieve your desired results. The good news here is that the attributes fueling your underlying operating system are the strings of the marionette that is you. Practice pulling the right string at the right time, and you will feel the freedom that comes from synching up your current and future selves.

COURAGE

Courage is your best defense against the discomforts of change. Tolerating change requires a whole lot of letting go . . . letting go of old, limiting beliefs, letting go of your larger pants size, tolerating improvement, understanding that hunger is not an emergency, and recognizing that true physical training is a privilege, not a burden, despite the challenges.

You must develop the courage to turn toward past discomforts. It's time to stop tolerating your being upset about the results that you didn't get from the actions you weren't courageous enough to take.

Without fear, there is no courage. To amplify your courage, you must embrace your fear, welcoming it with open arms. Let's recognize that fear is not the enemy; instead, it provides us with fertile soil for nurturing courage. So often when people talk about fear, they focus on the fight, flight, or freeze response. In *The Upside of Stress*, Kelly McGonigal lays out two other major stress responses worthy of attention, both of which will help you move forward toward health: (1) courage and (2) tend and befriend. Leveraging both will help you move from natural, primal instinct responses to more mature and adaptive approaches to fear.[8] **The very thing that you are avoiding is often where your power lies. This includes both thoughts and behaviors.**

To help you work on constructively facing your fear, let's break down the fight, flight, or freeze alternatives. The most aggressive of these is the courage response, which involves reinterpreting the inner sensations that you would normally label as stress. For example, think of the butterflies in your stomach before you embark on some new challenge. Instead of interpreting this feeling as negative, reimagine those butterflies in attack formation, preparing to help you slay whatever has prompted your nervousness! Practice seeing yourself as the victor you wish to become. Think less and execute more. Throw on some intense music and settle into that future self you know you can be.

The other fear response that can help you achieve your goals is tend and befriend. Here the key is to reach out to your community for help. Are you afraid you will fail? Get a teammate on board. Call a friend and tell them where your head is. Commit publicly to your goals and ask for support. You'll find power in community by teaming up with others. Or work to support someone else in similar endeavors. Often we follow through on a promise to others faster than we do for ourselves. When you're feeling less than strong, draw upon the strength of those around you. Remember that a meaningful life is not a fearless one but a courageous one.

PERSEVERANCE

Perseverance is the ability to execute on a task or plan despite its difficulty or delayed gratification. Get clear on what you want to achieve. Your goals could be strength-, weight-, or longevity-related. They could include self-imposed hard physical challenges. But each must be defined by measurable targets.

Perseverance means acknowledging that you will fall, likely multiple times, but you will keep getting back up. Patience and self-compassion are mandatory for perseverance to do its magic.

We all go through periods when we struggle to execute the plan. Not long ago, when I was having a hard time living up to the commitments I had made to myself, I called my friend and trainer Kara Killian for help. Together we loaded up backpacks with fifty pounds each and set out to ruck for ten miles through the streets of New York City. A staple of military training, rucking is hiking while carrying a weighted pack. Kara and I did this in winter and summer, rain or shine. This SUCKED! But we did it anyway, simply to build perseverance. I wanted to quit the first fifteen times, and then something magical happened. I embraced the suck of it all. I experienced the perseverance that's critical to merging your present and future selves. That awareness helped me persist through mile after sucky mile.

SELF-DISCIPLINE

While discipline is externally regulated, self-discipline relies on internal oversight. It's all about resisting temptations, controlling emotions, and overcoming weaknesses. We have all known highly disciplined people who are successful in terms of finances, friends, and family yet lack the self-discipline to consistently take the steps necessary for their health.

The quickest way to improve self-discipline is to plan for your weaknesses. Don't allow yourself to be surprised by your own human nature. You know your typical failure points; I guarantee it. Where does your self-discipline drop out? When someone brings sweets to the office? When you reach for a glass of wine after work, telling yourself tomorrow will be the day you'll stop? Without planning strategies for outwitting your human nature, you'll wind up chasing short-term pleasure/relief/gratification over long-term health. The fastest way to overcome this self-defeating cycle is to implement consequences in advance. The right penalty will help you meet your objectives.

One patient of mine went foraging through her kitchen every night after her husband and children went to bed. Not until she held herself accountable did she finally quit late-night snacking. She decided that the next time she broke her promise to herself, she'd have to jump into the cold ocean near her house. It took just one frigid dip for her to learn how to uphold her commitment.

ADAPTABILITY

Controlling your environment can help you prioritize and plan for proper nutrition and exercise. But if you live in the real world, you know all too well what happens to the best-laid plans . . . To combat the inevitable unpredictability in life, prepare yourself to shift gears using your powers of adaptability.

Here's an example from my own life. When my career started demanding more and more travel, I wound up eating and training a bit haphazardly, which slowly eroded my confidence in myself and my sense of personal integrity. If I couldn't keep my routines intact, how could I expect that of my patients?

Now, before departure, I research local gyms to find out what equipment they have. I also plot my training time into my travel schedule. My commitment to working out at those times is nonnegotiable. Whether or not I want to that day, I train according to my plan. Travel days can make me hungry. I often wake up too early after a night of poor sleep. Knowing that all these factors have the potential to erode my willpower, I plan for them in advance. I bring along beef jerky, protein bars, or a low-carb snack to eat en route. When the plane lands, I head straight to a grocery store to pick up the food I'll need during my stay and for the trip home.

Routine disruptions call upon us to adapt. I used to let the idea of perfect execution get in the way of adaptability, but by now I've done enough internal work to strategize around my own personal pitfalls. You can do this, too! Work-arounds are even more essential now that I'm a parent. Adaptability is 100 percent necessary for those of us caring for others, because caretaking is filled with unexpected situations that require us to pivot. Sick child keeping you from the gym? Time to break out that home workout you have on tap for interruptions like this. Even a set of resistance bands and maybe a couple of kettlebells can give you the tools you need to stick with your training goals for the day. When the unexpected derails your plans, make the commitment to yourself that you will be willing to find a solution rather than an excuse.

Perfectionistic ideals are a slippery slope, especially when it comes to wellness plans. Adaptability is your best defense.

- Out to dinner at a restaurant that can't accommodate the precise meal from your nutrition plan? Make the wisest choices you can from what's available.
- All the gyms closed during your beach stay? Pack up some sandbags to use as weights.
- Roads too snowy to make it to the gym? Time to get out that shovel or fill some garbage bags to get in some lifting.

The only limit to finding ways to achieve your goals is a lack of imagination. There are a million ways to execute your plan.

RESILIENCE

Resilience is the ability to return to baseline after a setback. This tricky yet essential trait involves cultivating your emotional intelligence. And as any human can tell you, emotions are messy.

Over and over, I have seen individuals fall off the wellness wagon when faced with a life challenge and never get back on. Disruptions come in all shapes and sizes. Some constitute overt crises, while others stem from subtle insults to our daily emotional well-being based on our interpretations of the world around us. I've found that the key to successfully returning to your baseline is to do so quickly.

Maybe a vacation, an illness, an injury, or some other interruption to your routine sets you back, and you fall out of rhythm. This moment can leave you extremely vulnerable to defeatist thoughts that can easily fuel self-defeating behaviors. The faster you get back to an empowered emotional state, the higher you are on the resiliency spectrum and the more successful you will be at reaching your goals.

For example, maybe after finally reaching your body composition goals, you return from a month of travel to realize you've gained back all the fat you lost. You didn't plan for this. What now?

A partner can help. Know whom you can call to have your back, then reach out right away to avoid wasting time feeling bad about yourself. Instead, make a game plan for how to move forward to get back in alignment with your self-standards. I recently called my longtime wingman Peter Roth to help get me back on track with executing for the future rather than moping about the past. "Let's add two extra workout days," I told him.

"Meet me outside at 6:45 a.m. five days a week so we can train." My next call was to my epic friend Roxy who brings me positive energy. I told her my diet and training commitments, and we checked in each day. I shared with her my future self as if my present self had already arrived at the place I wanted to end up.

Another fast-track way to increase resilience is to add in humor. In all things, vitamin H can be a super supplement. The humor you find in a tricky situation can lessen the blow and help you regulate your emotions. For example, remember my Navy SEAL patient, Brian? Whenever he spoke about his leg, he joked about how, for the rest of his life, buying shoes would cost him double because he'd have to pay for two instead of one. Recognizing how incredibly disempowering negative thoughts are, resilient individuals will find creative ways to switch their mindset from victim to victor, and fast. The best part about vitamin H is that it's not a hard pill to swallow. Do you find humor in life's upsets or take yourself too seriously? If you're having trouble joking about yourself, give me a call, and I will help!

The second most effective way to return to your baseline is to snap yourself out of negativity. If you cannot do this by reining in your thoughts, your body can help. All it takes is a few intervals of running or bike sprints, push-ups, sit-ups, or air squats for time. This allows you to use your body to control your mind. When you push your body hard into the zone of fatigue, you'll find you're no longer fighting against yourself. Instead, you recognize the freedom you have to choose what you think. If you cannot move your mind, move your body instead.

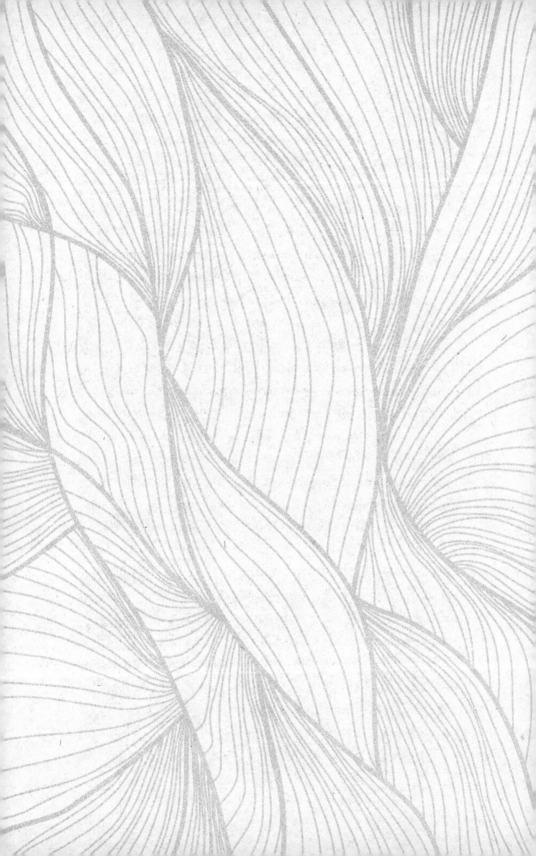

10.

~~~~~~~

Now, You Take the Reins

MAXIMIZE YOUR ENVIRONMENT

Now that you have your nutrition and training plans, how can you make them stick?

Identifying your personal relationship with external stimulus and influence can help you motivate your present self to take steps toward becoming your future self. By creating a targeted environment with triggers that elicit positive behaviors, discourage negative behaviors, and help you maintain momentum, you can create habits of health that allow for excellence.

- Post visual reminders of the goals you want to achieve, quotes that inspire mental toughness, or the attributes that you wish to embody.
- Put your training gear in places that will spur you to get up and go.
- Get ready for a morning workout by sleeping in your exercise clothes.

■ Remove tempting, but unhelpful, foods and clutter from your environment.

These are just a few examples of bulletproofing your physical space and creating the circumstances to generate positive actions.

Environmental Design—Accountability—Social Support
Create the space that is conducive to your success and allows you to execute, even on your worst days.

When it comes to physical training, choose the environment that will encourage you to put in maximum effort for maximum results. It helps to identify your domain of flow. Typically speaking, I find that people fall into one of the following categories.

1. **The Performer.** You don't train well alone. You may not need someone watching you throughout your workout, but you will train your hardest in an environment where there are other people, and you will be seen. You typically thrive in team sports or team-training scenarios such as CrossFit, group-training classes, or working one-on-one with a trainer. Many performer types who train solo end up with less-than-ideal results. You're less likely to push yourself, which leaves you open to subpar gym performance where you're just going through the motions. If you perform better with an audience, why not acknowledge that and use it to your advantage? In my case, I knew I needed a great gym environment after giving birth to my second child.

I'd learned after my first that I would need some hand-holding postpartum. (I still need that!) So I stick with the environment that pushes me to peak performance.

2. **The Solo Act.** These folks require no outside stimulus. This is a hard-charging, internally motivated group. For them, training is often meditative and therapeutic. They often don't need loud music or require anyone around them. In fact, they may find it distracting. Sound like you?

3. **The Chameleon.** Chameleons can push themselves in any environment, training with or without others. Many of those in the health and wellness space are chameleons. You can drop them into any situation, and they will perform. My dear friend Don Saladino is an example of this. You ask him at the last minute to go for a run, and he's there. Group training? No problem. These folks will show up and get the job done.

4. **The Reluctant.** Maybe you're a person who needs more privacy. Do you prefer not to exercise in front of others but still need external stimulation? Maybe a VRWorkout will provide the fun music, cool games, and privacy you need to push yourself. Or perhaps you could use a wall-mounted workout mirror that offers real-time feedback about form and intensity. One example is the Tonal mirror, which is designed to give you a complete strength workout with more than two hundred exercises to choose from. The system uses two built-in resistance arms with electromagnetic resistance to increase the weight of the cables up to 200 pounds.

Daily life offers plenty of distractions that can derail you into making excuses to miss your workouts. Take advantage of cues in your environment that will reinforce the message that this training—critical as it is for reaching your goals—is NONNEGOTIABLE.

Choose Your Hard

Far too often, and usually without much thought, people default into taking the easiest path. Choosing to do things the least difficult way is what we are programmed to do. It's part of who we are—or maybe who we have become. Unfortunately, doing what's convenient right now is no lasting strategy. It merely makes things more difficult later on . . . in virtually all cases. Instead of always looking for the path of least resistance, try choosing to do the hard things in life. That's what makes us strong.

Muscle-Centric Medicine® offers a new frame of reference for understanding exceptional health, flourishing through the aging process, and acknowledging muscle as the largest endocrine organ in the human body. Muscle health is the pinnacle, the missing ingredient, the scaffolding that supports the structures and ties together all the elements of longevity.

As I pored over mounds of research literature in the process of bringing this book to you, it became so apparent and unambiguous that medicine centers obesity as the first chapter of declining health. Obesity is not the beginning. It is just another disease land mine no different from or more or less important than other diseases.

The way of the future, Muscle-Centric Medicine® empowers us to return to the roots of our human design. These roots are grounded in physical strength and capability as well as the mental fortitude to navigate our weaknesses and any social or situational pressures we may face. We no longer confront physical predators; we face mental ones. We are up against an onslaught of media, agendas, and social-media influences, too many of which distort and distract from the real information that will make a difference in our lives and the lives of the people we love.

While the Lyon Protocol requires attention and effort, **it is much more difficult to live out the current model of predictable decline.** The Lyon Protocol calls upon us to rebalance ourselves and recalibrate the trajectory of life and death. The window of youth closes for all of us, as does the opportunity to fulfill our physical potential.

I made it my life's mission to help you. Teaching the truth about muscle as an organ, navigating nutrition, mastering your mind, and triumphing through physical training—these are vehicles that I can leverage to move you in the correct direction. We've reached the proverbial fork in the road.

Relieving suffering is what drives physicians to their work. Far too often in our culture, suffering comes as the slow, yet predictable, consequence of not taking care of one's body. For you, this changes today. Whether you come to this information as a physician, a coach, or simply a person interested in wellness, this book will stand by your side with the information and encouragement you have needed to support you in making real change.

Exceptional living and the ability to stand up and contribute to society, family, and community begin at the fundamental level of the physical. It exists at the base of the hierarchy of greatness. Exceptional living and contribution start with exceptional health.

The Lyon Protocol is a transformation journey. It has been my goal to serve as your guide, leading you out of the confusion, false narratives, and habits of mind and body that keep you shackled to mediocre well-being—or worse.

Lifestyle medicine is the tool I have used for more than a decade to help perpetuate real life transformation. And remember, how you do one thing is how you do all things. Building a plan and working *both* your skeletal muscle and your integrity muscle are skills translatable to living the life of your dreams.

You are the visionary for your own health journey. You will become the person you are meant to be. There is no time like now, so go out and seize what you deserve. Life offers no do-overs or repeats. The Lyon Protocol is the ultimate insurance policy, determining how you go through your life and how you glide into your last decades.

Now, for the grand finale, here are my best tips for getting yourself to work out and eat well consistently:

- Do not depend on motivation. Motivation ebbs and flows. It doesn't give you the consistency needed to garner success in the gym, the kitchen, or life.
- Motivation is rarely present when you're entering an uncomfortable realm—but that realm is precisely where growth occurs.
- Instead, focus on developing a new identity. This will give you the right mental framework to overcome obstacles, no matter the difficulty.

WHAT IF I FALL OFF?

Don't be an asshole to yourself; it is done. In my practice, I have seen patients continue to beat themselves up daily for falling off their plan. This never ends well. Buddhist teachings give us the concept of the second arrow. The first arrow is the initial experience of pain from a failing, a slight, or an attack. Sometimes this first arrow is self-inflicted, other times not. Either way, life comes with first arrows. That's just the way it is.

The second arrow, on the other hand, is the one you can control. That is the one you jab into yourself in the form of negative self-talk, globalizing, self-blame, "poor me" narratives, or any number of other scripts that we so often jump into following a painful occurrence.

I say, when that first painful arrow comes, pull it out. Fast. Don't shoot yourself with another. There is no need to compound the pain. What happened has happened. Take a moment to remember all the decisive steps you've already taken in your life that felt impossible at the time. Then remind yourself that you've tackled much harder situations, yet here you are. You will get back up again. And this time, I'll be at your side.

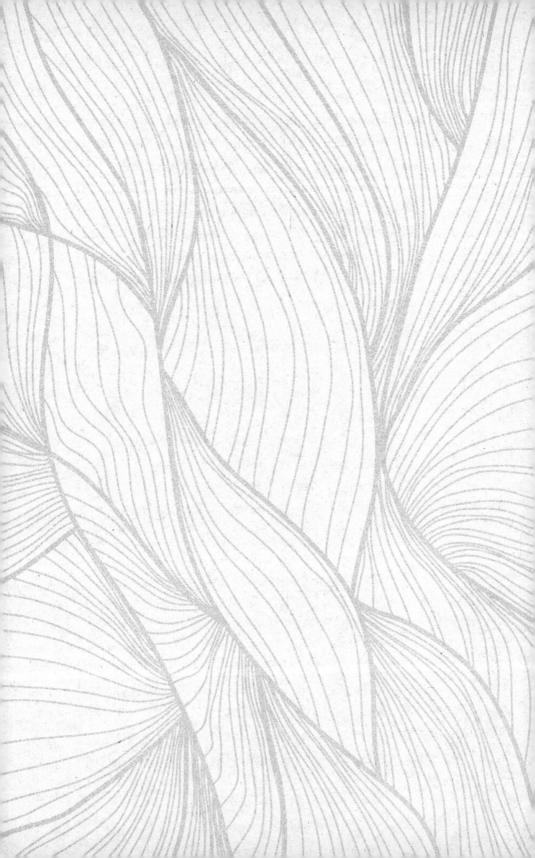

ACKNOWLEDGMENTS

〰〰〰

S o many people made this book happen by supporting me in all domains of life. This list is not exhaustive as there are so many to mention; included are a handful.

Don Layman, you have made such an impact on our world. Your research on protein has set a new standard for what optimal health looks like. Without you, Muscle-Centric Medicine® would not exist. I'm beyond grateful for our friendship, your mentorship, and the honor of collaborating and spreading this work in the world.

Liz Lipski, my godmother, you are all that and more. You introduced me to the world of medicine and nutrition. I have my roots and wings because of you.

To my husband, best friend, and father of our two children, Aries and Leonidas, former Navy SEAL Shane Kronstedt: You inspire me daily and have taught me that a teddy bear is still a bear. You are the foundation of excellence that we can all aspire to be. I love you. Aries and Leo, I strive to leave the world better because of you.

Peter Roth, your unwavering dedication to me, our family, and the mission is undeniable and irreplaceable. You have watched and believed by my side for more than a decade. You have a place in all our hearts.

Alexia Belrose, my assistant and teammate, I'm grateful you decided to take a chance on a new career. Without you, none of this would have been possible. You show up, execute, and are relentless in helping me. I am lucky to have you on my team.

Madeleine Novich, my sister and life wingman, I love you and couldn't ask for a more noble woman and sounding board in my life.

To my mother, Lennie Rose, I have the high standards and discipline because of you. No doubt, I would not be where I am had you not been my mother.

To Nathan Resnick, my father and always a best friend, I'm glad my career as a flight attendant didn't work out. Thank you for allowing me the freedom to explore and the fearless nature you instilled in me.

Uncle Howard and Aunt Ilene, you both saw my path before I did. You were always there encouraging me over a lifetime. Nothing I have done has been easy, and you always listened through tears of frustration and now gratitude. Thank you for being there from the beginning.

Kara K. Lazauskas, you are family. Our lives have never been the same since you. A true ride-or-die, you are something extraordinary. Thank you for being so deeply involved in our lives and hearts.

Ghena Grinsphun, my best friend and godfather to our kids, you are one in a million. Thank you for loving me as I am, with no judgment, and for years. You are brilliant, and your brilliance is only overshadowed by your heart.

Theresa Depasquale, my children's godmother, and sister, I love you to the moon and back. Thank you for being fierce in having my back, being in all the ups and downs with me, and always showing up. You are our extended family from beginning to end. You see the best in me and always provide vision and guidance on what is coming. Most important, you always pick up the incessant FaceTime calls from OUR kids.

Don Saladino, you are the most giving human I have ever met. Your energy is contagious, and, most important, you show up. I know there isn't anything you would not do for us and vice versa. You are my brother and inspiration, both personally and professionally. We love you and Mel and the family. Thank you for always telling it to me straight. I am a better communicator and doctor because of you.

Ralph Esposito, you are a superstar. Thank you for being on our squad, truthful, clear, and brilliant. You are wise and a force to be reckoned with. Thank you for listening and contributing to ideas, science, and friendship.

Elena Brower, my sister, thank you for showing me what is possible, freeing, and true, for listening and hearing all these years.

Anthony Lyon, thank you for being the springboard. I have learned so much from you.

Jim Kochalka, without you, my headspace would have self-imploded, guaranteed. I have learned so much from you about navigating the best version of myself. Thank you for always making time. You have opened my eyes to myself, and I am fortunate for the friendship.

Alexis Cowan, my bestie immediately, you are brilliant, and I appreciate and love you for helping me change the world.

To my brothers in science and medicine Alan Aragon and Ted Naiman, thank you for letting me call you, having intellectual integrity, and being all-around great humans. You are both so wise and gracious.

Emily Frisella, you inspire me daily with your capacity and work ethic. I'm even more impressed with the person you are. You make the chop-wood, carry-water grind more fun, and I am so grateful for the friendship. So many long days and nights, and you have come in strong with the humor game. I feel like someone "gets me." It's not about the work but about the contributions to make, and no one understands that more than you.

Malty Maharaj, thank you for keeping our lives and our kids together. You are a joy, and I'm so grateful you came into our lives. This book would have been impossible without your help.

Bedros Keuilian, you show me what right looks like. You are an incredible human, with character and charisma for days. Thanks to you and Diana for making us feel like family, for helping me trust myself in business and develop courage outside of the lane of caring for people and exemplifying servant leadership.

Jessica DuLong, you are the ultimate professional, making magic with this book despite everything. You are amazing.

Joy Tutela, thank you for going to bat and believing in me. I hope this is one of many.

Beth Lipton, thank you for making the introductions that birthed this book and for the attention to the recipes.

To all my patients and to you, the reader, thank you for being the reason this exists.

APPENDIX

~~~~~~

MEAL PLANS AND RECIPES

OPTIMIZE LONGEVITY PLAN
Three meals a day

MEAL 1

SHAKE + EGGS
Purple Magic Shake (page 348) — *27 g protein, 22 g carbs, 13 g fat, 6 g fiber*
3 hard-cooked large eggs — *18 g protein, 0 g carbs, 15 g fat, 0 g fiber*
1 hard-cooked large egg white — *4 g protein, 0 g carbs, 0 g fat, 0 g fiber*
1 Wasa cracker — *1 g protein, 10 g carbs, 0 g fat, 2 g fiber*
                    Total — **580 calories, 50 g protein, 32 g carbs, 28 g fat, 8 g fiber**

DENVER SCRAMBLE
1 teaspoon avocado oil — *0 g protein, 0 g carbs, 5 g fat, 0 g fiber*
¼ cup chopped onion — *0 g protein, 4 g carbs, 0 g fat, 1 g fiber*
½ cup chopped bell pepper — *1 g protein, 5 g carbs, 0 g fat, 2 g fiber*
2 ounces Canadian bacon — *16 g protein, 1 g carbs, 2 g fat, 0 g fiber*
3 large eggs — *18 g protein, 2 g carbs, 16 g fat, 0 g fiber*
3 large egg whites — *12 g protein, 1 g carbs, 0 g fat, 0 g fiber*
1 Wasa cracker — *1 g protein, 10 g carbs, 0 g fat, 2 g fiber*
½ cup berries — *1 g protein, 11 g carbs, 0 g fat, 2 g fiber*
                    Total — **539 calories, 49 g protein, 34 g carbs, 23 g fat, 7 g fiber**

*In a large skillet, heat the oil over medium-high heat. Add the onion and
bell pepper and cook until softened, 4 to 5 minutes. Add the Canadian
bacon; sauté until lightly golden. Add the eggs and whites; cook until the
desired doneness. Enjoy the cracker and berries on the side.*

CHIA PUDDING

½ cup plain low-fat Greek yogurt — *13 g protein, 5 g carbs, 2 g fat, 0 g fiber*
½ cup water
1¼ scoops whey protein powder — *30 g protein, 2 g carbs, 1 g fat, 0 g fiber*
2 tablespoons chia seeds — *3 g protein, 8 g carbs, 6 g fat, 7 g fiber*
Pinch of salt
⅛ teaspoon cinnamon, optional
⅛ teaspoon vanilla extract, optional
1 cup berries — *1 g protein, 21 g carbs, 1 g fat, 4 g fiber*
1 teaspoon sliced almonds — *1 g protein, 0 g carbs, 1 g fat, 0 g fiber*

Total — **435 calories, 48 g protein, 36 g carbs, 11 g fat, 11 g fiber**

Combine the yogurt, water, protein powder, chia seeds, and salt in a small bowl. Stir in the cinnamon and/or vanilla, if using. Top with the berries and almonds.

MEAL 2

TURKEY CLUB LETTUCE WRAPS

¼ cup mashed avocado — *1 g protein, 5 g carbs, 9 g fat, 4 g fiber*
2 teaspoons pesto — *1 g protein, 0 g carbs, 4 g fat, 0 g fiber*
3 large romaine leaves — *1 g protein, 3 g carbs, 0 g fat, 2 g fiber*
¼ cup chopped cherry tomatoes — *0 g protein, 2 g carbs, 0 g fat, 1 g fiber*
4 ounces organic roasted turkey (such as Applegate) — *20 g protein, 0 g carbs, 0 g fat, 0 g fiber*
½ cup berries — *1 g protein, 11 g carbs, 0 g fat, 2 g fiber*

Total — **297 calories, 24 g protein, 21 g carbs, 13 g fat, 9 g fiber**

Spread the avocado and pesto in the lettuce leaves. Divide the tomatoes and turkey among the leaves; roll up and eat. Enjoy the berries for dessert.

SHRIMP STIR-FRY

1½ teaspoons avocado oil — *0 g protein, 0 g carbs, 7 g fat, 0 g fiber*

4 ounces shrimp, peeled and deveined — *18 g protein, 0 g carbs, 1 g fat, 0 g fiber*

1 tablespoon coconut aminos — *0 g protein, 3 g carbs, 0 g fat, 0 g fiber*

1 serving Stir-Fried Vegetables (page 330) — *5 g protein, 15 g carbs, 10 g fat, 4 g fiber*

Total — 353 calories, 23 g protein, 18 g carbs, 21 g fat, 4 g fiber

Heat the oil in a medium skillet over medium-high heat. Add the shrimp and cook until they have turned pink, about 2 minutes; season with the coconut aminos. Serve with the vegetables.

TUNA + BEET SALAD

1 serving Shredded Beet and Carrot Salad (page 334) — *2 g protein, 12 g carbs, 8 g fat, 3 g fiber*

½ can (5 ounces) light tuna packed in olive oil, drained — *18 g protein, 0 g carbs, 5 g fat, 0 g fiber*

1 Wasa cracker — *1 g protein, 10 g carbs, 0 g fat, 2 g fiber*

Total — 289 calories, 21 g protein, 22 g carbs, 13 g fat, 5 g fiber

MEAL 3

STEAK + VEG + RICE

1 serving Pan-Seared Flank Steak (page 305) — *37 g protein, 0 g carbs, 14 g fat, 0 g fiber*

1 serving Braised Radicchio and Endive (page 338) — *8 g protein, 23 g carbs, 5 g fat, 14 g fiber*

1 serving Bone Broth Rice (page 331) — *4 g protein, 22 g carbs, 0 g fat, 0 g fiber*

Total — 547 calories, 49 g protein, 45 g carbs, 19 g fat, 14 g fiber

BUFFALO CHICKEN SALAD

5 ounces cooked chicken breast — *43 g protein, 0 g carbs, 4 g fat, 0 g fiber*

3 ribs celery, minced — *1 g protein, 4 g carbs, 0 g fat, 2 g fiber*

2 medium carrots, minced — *1 g protein, 12 g carbs, 0 g fat, 3 g fiber*

1½ tablespoons avocado oil mayonnaise — *0 g protein, 0 g carbs, 18 g fat, 0 g fiber*

1½ tablespoons Frank's RedHot (or other buffalo sauce) — *1 g protein, 0 g carbs, 0 g fat, 0 g fiber*

2 cups chopped mixed greens — *1 g protein, 2 g carbs, 0 g fat, 1 g fiber*

1 medium apple — *1 g protein, 25 g carbs, 0 g fat, 4 g fiber*

Total — 558 calories, 48 g protein, 43 g carbs, 22 g fat, 10 g fiber

Combine the chicken, celery, carrots, mayonnaise, and hot sauce in a medium bowl; fold together. Serve on the mixed greens. Enjoy an apple for dessert.

TACO STUFFED PEPPERS

1 serving Taco Stuffed Peppers (page 309) — *36 g protein, 17 g carbs, 13 g fat, 5 g fiber*

½ cup plain low-fat Greek yogurt — *13 g protein, 5 g carbs, 2 g fat, 0 g fiber*

1 teaspoon honey — *0 g protein, 6 g carbs, 0 g fat, 0 g fiber*

1 cup berries — *1 g protein, 21 g carbs, 1 g fat, 4 g fiber*

Total — 540 calories, 50 g protein, 49 g carbs, 16 g fat, 9 g fiber

Bonus for dessert *— Mix the yogurt with the honey; top with the berries.*

COD WITH BAKED POTATO

1 serving Walnut-Crusted Cod (page 325) — *33 g protein, 3 g carbs, 15 g fat, 1 g fiber*

1 medium baked potato (with skin) — *4 g protein, 37 g carbs, 0 g fat, 4 g fiber*

2 tablespoons plain low-fat Greek yogurt — *3 g protein, 1 g carbs, 1 g fat, 0 g fiber*

3 slices bacon — *8 g protein, 0 g carbs, 8 g fat, 0 g fiber*

Olive or avocado oil cooking spray

1 cup chopped broccoli — *3 g protein, 6 g carbs, 0 g fat, 2 g fiber*

1 teaspoon lemon pepper seasoning — *0 g protein, 1 g carbs, 0 g fat, 0 g fiber*

Total — 612 calories, 51 g protein, 48 g carbs, 24 g fat, 7 g fiber

Serve the cod with the baked potato topped with the yogurt and crumbled bacon. Mist a small skillet with cooking spray and cook the broccoli over medium-high heat, until crisp-tender, 4 to 5 minutes. Season with the lemon pepper or other seasoning.

OPTIMIZE QUALITY WEIGHT LOSS PLAN
Three meals a day plus optional snack after Meal 3

MEAL 1

PROTEIN SHAKE
1 scoop whey protein powder — *24 g protein, 2 g carbs, 1 g fat, 0 g fiber*
½ cup plain low-fat Greek yogurt — *13 g protein, 5 g carbs, 2 g fat, 0 g fiber*
1 cup berries — *1 g protein, 21 g carbs, 0 g fat, 4 g fiber*
1 tablespoon MCT oil — *0 g protein, 0 g carbs, 14 g fat, 0 g fiber*
1 teaspoon vanilla extract — *0 g protein, 1 g carbs, 0 g fat, 0 g fiber*
Water
            Total — **421 calories, 38 g protein, 29 g carbs, 17 g fat, 4 g fiber**

BURGER + EGGS
2 hard-cooked (steamed) large eggs — *12 g protein, 1 g carbs, 11 g fat, 0 g fiber*
1 hard-cooked large egg white — *4 g protein, 0 g carbs, 0 g fat, 0 g fiber*
½ Herbed Burger patty (page 311) — *21 g protein, 0 g carbs, 5 g fat, 1 g fiber*
1¼ cups berries — *1 g protein, 27 g carbs, 1 g fat, 5 g fiber*
            Total — **417 calories, 38 g protein, 28 g carbs, 17 g fat, 6 g fiber**

CHIA PUDDING
½ cup plain low-fat Greek yogurt — *13 g protein, 5 g carbs, 2 g fat, 0 g fiber*
¼ cup water
1 scoop whey protein powder — *24 g protein, 2 g carbs, 1 g fat, 0 g fiber*
2 tablespoons chia seeds — *3 g protein, 8 g carbs, 6 g fat, 7 g fiber*

Pinch of salt

⅛ teaspoon cinnamon, optional

⅛ teaspoon vanilla extract, optional

¾ cup berries — *1 g protein, 16 g carbs, 0 g fat, 3 g fiber*

1 teaspoon sliced almonds — *1 g protein, 0 g carbs, 1 g fat, 0 g fiber*

Total — 382 calories, 42 g protein, 31 g carbs, 10 g fat, 10 g fiber

Combine the yogurt, water, protein powder, chia seeds, and salt in a small bowl. Stir in the cinnamon and/or vanilla, if using. Top with the berries and almonds.

MEAL 2

Or optional snack: 10–20 g protein, < 10 g carbs (string cheese or meat stick, no sugar).

GREEN GODDESS COBB SALAD

1 serving Green Goddess Cobb Salad (page 315) — *33 g protein, 8 g carbs, 13 g fat, 4 g fiber*

1 tablespoon extra dressing — *0 g protein, 1 g carbs, 4 g fat, 1 g fiber*

2 Wasa crackers — *3 g protein, 20 g carbs, 1 g fat, 4 g fiber*

Total — 422 calories, 36 g protein, 29 g carbs, 18 g fat, 9 g fiber

SHRIMP STIR-FRY

1½ teaspoons avocado oil — *0 g protein, 0 g carbs, 7 g fat, 0 g fiber*

5 ounces shrimp, peeled and deveined — *23 g protein, 0 g carbs, 1 g fat, 0 g fiber*

1 serving Stir-Fried Vegetables (page 330) — *5 g protein, 15 g carbs, 10 g fat, 4 g fiber*

½ serving Bone Broth Rice (page 331) — *2 g protein, 11 g carbs, 0 g fat, 0 g fiber*

Total — 386 calories, 30 g protein, 26 g carbs, 18 g fat, 4 g fiber

Heat the oil in a medium skillet over medium-high heat. Add the shrimp and cook until they have turned pink, about 2 minutes. Serve with the vegetables and rice.

BURGER + RICE

1 serving Bone Broth Rice (page 331) — *4 g protein, 22 g carbs, 0 g fat, 0 g fiber*

½ Herbed Burger patty (page 311) — *21 g protein, 0 g carbs, 5 g fat, 1 g fiber*

½ ounce sharp cheddar — *3 g protein, 1 g carbs, 5 g fat, 0 g fiber*

½ avocado — *1 g protein, 6 g carbs, 11 g fat, 5 g fiber*

Total — **421 calories, 29 g protein, 29 g carbs, 21 g fat, 6 g fiber**

PORK + SWEET POTATOES

1 serving Garlic Rosemary Roast Pork Tenderloin (page 317) — *30 g protein, 1 g carbs, 7 g fat, 0 g fiber*

½ serving Mashed Purple Sweet Potatoes with Sesame (page 337) — *2 g protein,19 g carbs, 3 g fat, 3 g fiber*

1 serving Tangy Coleslaw (page 336) — *1 g protein, 7 g carbs, 7 g fat, 2 g fiber*

Total — **393 calories, 33 g protein, 27 g carbs, 17 g fat, 5 g fiber**

TUNA + BEET SALAD

1 serving Shredded Beet and Carrot Salad (page 334) — *2 g protein, 12 g carbs, 8 g fat, 3 g fiber*

1½ tablespoons hemp seeds — *5 g protein, 2 g carbs, 8 g fat, 1 g fiber*

½ can (5 ounces) light tuna packed in olive oil, drained — *18 g protein, 0 g carbs, 5 g fat, 0 g fiber*

½ cup berries — *1 g protein, 11 g carbs, 0 g fat, 2 g fiber*

Total — **393 calories, 26 g protein, 25 g carbs, 21 g fat, 6 g fiber**

STEAK + GREEN BEANS

1 serving Pan-Seared Flank Steak (page 305) — *37 g protein, 0 g carbs, 14 g fat, 0 g fiber*

1 serving Green Beans and Shallots with Almonds (page 327) — *5 g protein, 15 g carbs, 8 g fat, 6 g fiber*

¾ cup berries — *1 g protein, 16 g carbs, 0 g fat, 3 g fiber*

Total — **494 calories, 43 g protein, 31 g carbs, 22 g fat, 9 g fiber**

MEAL 3

Optional post-meal snack: ½ cup berries (or other low-sugar fruit)

BURGER + RICE

1 serving Bone Broth Rice (page 331) — *4 g protein, 22 g carbs, 0 g fat, 0 g fiber*

1 Herbed Burger patty (page 311) — *42 g protein, 1 g carbs, 10 g fat, 2 g fiber*

½ avocado — *1 g protein, 6 g carbs, 11 g fat, 5 g fiber*

Total — 498 calories, 47 g protein, 29 g carbs, 21 g fat, 7 g fiber

BUFFALO CHICKEN SALAD

4 ounces cooked chicken breast — *34 g protein, 0 g carbs, 4 g fat, 0 g fiber*

2 ribs celery, minced — *1 g protein, 2 g carbs, 0 g fat, 1 g fiber*

1 medium carrot, minced — *0 g protein, 6 g carbs, 0 g fat, 2 g fiber*

1 tablespoon avocado oil mayonnaise — *0 g protein, 0 g carbs, 12 g fat, 0 g fiber*

1 tablespoon Frank's RedHot (or other buffalo sauce) — *0 g protein, 0 g carbs, 0 g fat, 0 g fiber*

2 cups chopped mixed greens — *1 g protein, 2 g carbs, 0 g fat, 1 g fiber*

2 Wasa crackers — *3 g protein, 20 g carbs, 1 g fat, 4 g fiber*

Total — 433 calories, 39 g protein, 30 g carbs, 17 g fat, 8 g fiber

Combine the chicken, celery, carrots, mayonnaise, and hot sauce in a medium bowl; fold together. Serve on the mixed greens with the crackers on the side.

SHRIMP STIR-FRY

1½ teaspoons avocado oil — *0 g protein, 0 g carbs, 7 g fat, 0 g fiber*

8 ounces shrimp, peeled and deveined — *36 g protein, 0 g carbs, 4 g fat, 0 g fiber*

1 serving Stir-Fried Vegetables (page 330) — *5 g protein, 15 g carbs, 10 g fat, 4 g fiber*

½ serving Bone Broth Rice (page 331) — *2 g protein, 11 g carbs, 0 g fat, 0 g fiber*

Total — 465 calories, 43 g protein, 26 g carbs, 21 g fat, 4 g fiber

Heat the oil in a large skillet over medium-high heat. Add the shrimp and cook until they have turned pink, about 2 minutes. Serve with the vegetables and rice.

PORK + SWEET POTATOES

1 serving Garlic Rosemary Roast Pork Tenderloin (page 317) — *30 g protein, 1 g carbs, 7 g fat, 0 g fiber*

1 hard-cooked large egg — *6 g protein, 0 g carbs, 5 g fat, 0 g fiber*

½ serving Mashed Purple Sweet Potatoes with Sesame (page 337) — *2 g protein, 19 g carbs, 3 g fat, 3 g fiber*

1 serving Tangy Coleslaw (page 336) — *1 g protein, 7 g carbs, 7 g fat, 2 g fiber*

Total — 462 calories, 39 g protein, 27 g carbs, 22 g fat, 5 g fiber

SALMON + BEET SALAD

1 serving Shredded Beet and Carrot Salad (page 334) — *2 g protein, 12 g carbs, 8 g fat, 3 g fiber*

1 serving Poached Salmon (page 319) — *37 g protein, 0 g carbs, 14 g fat*

½ serving Bone Broth Rice (page 331) — *2 g protein, 11 g carbs, 0 g fat, 0 g fiber*

½ cup berries — *1 g protein, 11 g carbs, 0 g fat, 2 g fiber*

Total — 502 calories, 42 g protein, 34 g carbs, 22 g fat, 19 g fiber

STEAK + GREEN BEANS

1 serving Pan-Seared Flank Steak (page 305) — *37 g protein, 0 g carbs, 14 g fat, 0 g fiber*

1 serving Green Beans and Shallots with Almonds (page 327) — *5 g protein, 15 g carbs, 8 g fat, 6 g fiber*

¾ cup berries — *1 g protein, 16 g carbs, 0 g fat, 3 g fiber*

Total — 494 calories, 43 g protein, 31 g carbs, 22 g fat, 9 g fiber

OPTIMIZE MUSCLE PLAN
Four meals a day

MEAL 1

SHAKE + EGGS
Purple Magic Shake (page 348) — *27 g protein, 22 g carbs, 13 g fat, 6 g fiber*
3 hard-cooked large eggs — *18 g protein, 0 g carbs, 15 g fat, 0 g fiber*
1 hard-cooked large egg white — *4 g protein, 0 g carbs, 0 g fat, 0 g fiber*
                    Total — **536 calories, 49 g protein, 22 g carbs, 28 g fat, 6 g fiber**

CHIA PUDDING
½ cup plain low-fat Greek yogurt — *13 g protein, 5 g carbs, 2 g fat, 0 g fiber*
⅓ cup water
1¼ scoops whey protein powder — *30 g protein, 2 g carbs, 1 g fat, 0 g fiber*
2 tablespoons chia seeds — *3 g protein, 8 g carbs, 6 g fat, 7 g fiber*
Pinch of salt
⅛ teaspoon cinnamon, optional
⅛ teaspoon vanilla extract, optional
½ cup berries — *1 g protein, 11 g carbs, 0 g fat, 2 g fiber*
1 teaspoon sliced almonds — *1 g protein, 0 g carbs, 1 g fat, 0 g fiber*
                    Total — **390 calories, 49 g protein, 26 g carbs, 10 g fat, 9 g fiber**

Combine the yogurt, water, protein powder, chia seeds, and salt in a small bowl. Stir in the cinnamon and/or vanilla, if using. Top with the berries and almonds.

DENVER SCRAMBLE
1 teaspoon avocado oil — *0 g protein, 0 g carbs, 5 g fat, 0 g fiber*
¼ cup chopped onion — *0 g protein, 4 g carbs, 0 g fat, 1 g fiber*
½ cup chopped bell pepper — *1 g protein, 5 g carbs, 0 g fat, 2 g fiber*
2 ounces Canadian bacon — *16 g protein, 1 g carbs, 2 g fat, 0 g fiber*
3 large eggs — *18 g protein, 2 g carbs, 16 g fat, 0 g fiber*
3 large egg whites — *11 g protein, 1 g carbs, 0 g fat, 0 g fiber*

1 Wasa cracker — *1 g protein, 10 g carbs, 0 g fat, 2 g fiber*
½ cup berries — *1 g protein, 11 g carbs, 0 g fat, 2 g fiber*
Total — 535 calories, 48 g protein, 34 g carbs, 23 g fat, 7 g fiber

In a large skillet, heat the oil over high heat. Add the onion and bell pepper and cook until softened, 4 to 5 minutes. Add the Canadian bacon; sauté until lightly golden. Add the eggs and whites; cook until the desired doneness. Enjoy the cracker and berries on the side.

MEAL 2

SALMON + BEET SALAD + RICE

1 serving Poached Salmon (page 319) — *37 g protein, 0 g carbs, 14 g fat, 0 g fiber*
1 hard-cooked large egg white — *4 g protein, 0 g carbs, 0 g fat, 0 g fiber*
1 serving Shredded Beet and Carrot Salad (page 334) — *2 g protein, 12 g carbs, 8 g fat, 3 g fiber*
½ serving Bone Broth Rice (page 331) — *2 g protein, 11 g carbs, 0 g fat, 0 g fiber*
Total — 470 calories, 45 g protein, 23 g carbs, 22 g fat, 3 g fiber

SHRIMP STIR-FRY

8 ounces shrimp, peeled and deveined — *36 g protein, 0 g carbs, 4 g fat, 0 g fiber*
1 large egg — *6 g protein, 1 g carbs, 5 g fat, 0 g fiber*
1½ teaspoons avocado oil — *0 g protein, 0 g carbs, 7 g fat, 0 g fiber*
1 serving Stir-Fried Vegetables (page 330) — *5 g protein, 15 g carbs, 10 g fat, 4 g fiber*
½ serving Bone Broth Rice (page 331) — *2 g protein, 11 g carbs, 0 g fat, 0 g fiber*
Total — 538 calories, 49 g protein, 27 g carbs, 26 g fat, 4 g fiber

Heat the oil in a large skillet over medium-high heat. Add the shrimp and egg and cook, about 2 minutes. Serve with the vegetables and rice.

"SPAGHETTI" WITH MEAT SAUCE

2 cups spaghetti squash — *2 g protein, 20 g carbs, 1 g fat, 4 g fiber*

Olive or avocado oil cooking spray

Sea salt and freshly ground black pepper

1 serving Upgraded Ground Beef (page 308) — *46 g protein, 1 g carbs, 18 g fat, 0 g fiber*

½ cup no-sugar-added tomato sauce (such as Rao's) — *1 g protein, 3 g carbs, 5 g fat, 1 g fiber*

> *Total* — **508 calories, 49 g protein, 24 g carbs, 24 g fat, 5 g fiber**

Cut the squash in half crosswise, remove the seeds; mist with cooking spray, season with salt and pepper. Place the squash on a parchment-lined baking sheet; bake at 400°F until tender, about 25 minutes. Shred the squash into "noodles." Take out 2 cups; cover and refrigerate the rest. Mist a large skillet with cooking spray; cook the beef until cooked through. Add the sauce; simmer. Serve the sauce over the squash.

ROAST BEEF LETTUCE WRAPS

6 large romaine leaves — *2 g protein, 6 g carbs, 0 g fat, 4 g fiber*

1 tablespoon Dijon mustard — *1 g protein, 1 g carbs, 1 g fat, 1 g fiber*

6 ounces high-quality roast beef (such as Applegate Organics) — *40 g protein, 0 g carbs, 9 g fat, 0 g fiber*

1 ounce sharp cheddar — *6 g protein, 1 g carbs, 9 g fat, 1 g fiber*

¾ cup berries — *1 g protein, 16 g carbs, 0 g fat, 3 g fiber*

> *Total* — **467 calories, 50 g protein, 24 g carbs, 19 g fat, 9 g fiber**

Spread the romaine leaves with the mustard, then wrap the roast beef and cheddar in the leaves. Enjoy with the berries for dessert.

MEAL 3

ROAST BEEF LETTUCE WRAPS

6 large romaine leaves — *2 g protein, 6 g carbs, 0 g fat, 4 g fiber*

1 tablespoon Dijon mustard — *1 g protein, 1 g carbs, 1 g fat, 1 g fiber*

6 ounces high-quality roast beef (such as Applegate Organics) — *40 g protein, 0 g carbs, 9 g fat, 0 g fiber*

1 ounce sharp cheddar — *6 g protein, 1 g carbs, 9 g fat, 1 g fiber*
1¾ cups berries — *2 g protein, 38 g carbs, 0 g fat, 6 g fiber*
> *Total* — **478 calories, 51 g protein, 46 g carbs, 10 g fat, 12 g fiber**

Spread the romaine leaves with the mustard and wrap the roast beef and cheddar in the leaves. Enjoy with the berries for dessert.

PORK CHOP + VEG

1 "Perfect" Pork Chop (page 324) — *32 g protein, 0 g carbs, 17 g fat, 0 g fiber*
1 serving Roasted Brussels Sprouts, Carrots, and Onions (page 340) —
  6 g protein, 27 g carbs, 11 g fat, 9 g fiber
½ cup plain nonfat Greek yogurt — *13 g protein, 4 g carbs, 1 g fat, 0 g fiber*
½ cup berries — 1 g protein, 11 g carbs, 0 g fat, 2 g fiber
> *Total* — **637 calories, 52 g protein, 42 g carbs, 29 g fat, 11 g fiber**

BUFFALO CHICKEN SALAD

6 ounces cooked chicken breast — *51 g protein, 0 g carbs, 5 g fat, 0 g fiber*
3 ribs celery, minced — *1 g protein, 4 g carbs, 0 g fat, 2 g fiber*
2 medium carrots, minced — *1 g protein, 12 g carbs, 0 g fat, 3 g fiber*
1½ tablespoons avocado oil mayonnaise — *0 g protein, 0 g carbs, 18 g fat, 0 g fiber*
1½ tablespoons Frank's RedHot (or other buffalo sauce) — *1 g protein, 0 g carbs, 0 g fat, 0 g fiber*
2 cups chopped mixed greens — *1 g protein, 2 g carbs, 0 g fat, 1 g fiber*
1 large apple — *1 g protein, 31 g carbs, 0 g fat, 5 g fiber*
> *Total* — **623 calories, 56 g protein, 49 g carbs, 23 g fat, 11 g fiber**

Combine the chicken, celery, carrots, mayonnaise, and hot sauce in a medium bowl; fold together. Serve on the mixed greens. Enjoy an apple for dessert.

PORK LOIN + VEG

2 tablespoons plain low-fat Greek yogurt — *3 g protein, 1 g carbs, 1 g fat, 0 g fiber*
2 tablespoons jarred pesto — *2 g protein, 1 g carbs, 13 g fat, 0 g fiber*
1 small baked sweet potato — *2 g protein, 17 g carbs, 0 g fat, 3 g fiber*

1 serving Garlic Rosemary Pork Tenderloin (page 317) — *30 g protein, 1 g carbs, 7 g fat, 0 g fiber*

1 serving Braised Radicchio and Endive (page 338) — *8 g protein, 23 g carbs, 5 g fat, 14 g fiber*

Total — 586 calories, 45 g protein, 43 g carbs, 26 g fat, 17 g fiber

Mix the yogurt with the pesto in a small bowl and spoon it on top of the sweet potato. Enjoy with the pork and braised vegetables.

TUNA MELT

2 cauliflower sandwich thins (such as Outer Aisle) — *10 g protein, 2 g carbs, 6 g fat, 1 g fiber*

1 can (5 ounces) water-packed light tuna (drained) — *33 g protein, 0 g carbs, 1 g fat, 0 g fiber*

3 ribs celery, minced — *1 g protein, 4 g carbs, 0 g fat, 2 g fiber*

3 medium carrots, minced — *2 g protein, 18 g carbs, 0 g fat, 5 g fiber*

1 tablespoon avocado oil mayonnaise — *0 g protein, 0 g carbs, 12 g fat, 0 g fiber*

1 ounce sharp cheddar, shredded — *6 g protein, 1 g carbs, 9 g fat, 1 g fiber*

1 medium apple — *1 g protein, 25 g carbs, 0 g fat, 4 g fiber*

Total — 664 calories, 53 g protein, 50 g carbs, 28 g fat, 12 g fiber

Defrost the sandwich thins; lightly toast on a baking sheet at 350°F. Mix the tuna, celery, carrots, and mayonnaise. Scoop onto the sandwich thins. Sprinkle with the cheddar; broil until the cheese is melted and bubbly. Enjoy an apple for dessert.

COD WITH BAKED POTATO

1 serving Walnut-Crusted Cod (page 325) — *33 g protein, 3 g carbs, 15 g fat, 1 g fiber*

1 medium baked potato (with skin) — *4 g protein, 37 g carbs, 0 g fat, 4 g fiber*

2 tablespoons plain low-fat Greek yogurt — *3 g protein, 1 g carbs, 1 g fat, 0 g fiber*

3 slices bacon — *8 g protein, 0 g carbs, 8 g fat, 0 g fiber*

Olive or avocado oil cooking spray

1 cup chopped broccoli — *3 g protein, 6 g carbs, 0 g fat, 2 g fiber*
1 teaspoon lemon pepper seasoning — *0 g protein, 1 g carbs, 0 g fat,*
   0 g fiber
          Total *—* **612 calories, 51 g protein, 48 g carbs, 24 g fat, 7 g fiber**

Serve the cod with the baked potato topped with the yogurt and
crumbled bacon. Mist a small skillet with cooking spray and cook the
broccoli over medium-high heat, until crisp-tender, 4 to 5 minutes.
Season with the lemon pepper or other seasoning.

MEAL 4

PORK CHOP + VEG

1 "Perfect" Pork Chop (page 324) — *32 g protein, 0 g carbs, 17 g fat,*
   0 g fiber
1 serving Roasted Brussels Sprouts, Carrots, and Onions (page 340) —
   6 g protein, 27 g carbs, 11 g fat, 9 g fiber
½ cup plain nonfat Greek yogurt — *13 g protein, 4 g carbs, 1 g fat, 0 g fiber*
½ cup berries — *1 g protein, 11 g carbs, 0 g fat, 2 g fiber*
          Total *—* **637 calories, 52 g protein, 42 g carbs, 29 g fat, 11 g fiber**

BUFFALO CHICKEN SALAD

6 ounces cooked chicken breast — *51 g protein, 0 g carbs, 5 g fat, 0 g fiber*
3 ribs celery (minced) — *1 g protein, 4 g carbs, 0 g fat, 2 g fiber*
2 medium carrots, minced — *1 g protein, 12 g carbs, 0 g fat, 3 g fiber*
1½ tablespoons avocado oil mayonnaise — *0 g protein, 0 g carbs, 18 g fat,*
   0 g fiber
1½ tablespoons Frank's RedHot (or other buffalo sauce) — *1 g protein,*
   0 g carbs, 0 g fat, 0 g fiber
2 cups chopped mixed greens — *1 g protein, 2 g carbs, 0 g fat, 1 g fiber*
1 large apple — *1 g protein, 31 g carbs, 0 g fat, 5 g fiber*
          Total *—* **623 calories, 56 g protein, 49 g carbs, 23 g fat, 11 g fiber**

Combine the chicken, celery, carrots, mayonnaise, and hot sauce in a
medium bowl; fold together. Serve on the mixed greens. Enjoy an apple
for dessert.

PORK LOIN + VEG

2 tablespoons plain low-fat Greek yogurt — *3 g protein, 1 g carbs, 1 g fat, 0 g fiber*

2 tablespoons jarred pesto — *2 g protein, 1 g carbs, 13 g fat, 0 g fiber*

1 small baked sweet potato — *2 g protein, 17 g carbs, 0 g fat, 3 g fiber*

1 serving Garlic Rosemary Roast Pork Tenderloin (page 317) — *30 g protein, 1 g carbs, 7 g fat, 0 g fiber*

1 serving Braised Radicchio and Endive (page 338) — *8 g protein, 23 g carbs, 5 g fat, 14 g fiber*

Total — **586 calories, 45 g protein, 43 g carbs, 26 g fat, 17 g fiber**

Mix the yogurt with the pesto in a small bowl and spoon on top of the sweet potato. Enjoy with the pork and braised vegetables.

BURGER SALAD

1 serving Upgraded Ground Beef (page 308) — *46 g protein, 1 g carbs, 18 g fat, 0 g fiber*

2 cups chopped mixed greens — *1 g protein, 2 g carbs, 0 g fat, 1 g fiber*

2 medium carrots, minced — *1 g protein, 12 g carbs, 0 g fat, 3 g fiber*

2 Persian cucumbers, chopped — *0 g protein, 8 g carbs, 0 g fat, 2 g fiber*

1 tablespoon vinaigrette — *0 g protein, 1 g carbs, 6 g fat, 0 g fiber*

1 cup berries — *1 g protein, 21 g carbs, 0 g fat, 4 g fiber*

Total — **592 calories, 49 g protein, 45 g carbs, 24 g fat, 10 g fiber**

RECIPES

PAN-SEARED FLANK STEAK
(STEAK + VEG + RICE) (STEAK + GREEN BEANS)

Flank is a lean cut of steak, yet it has a lot of rich flavor. When cooked to medium-rare, it's tender and delicious. If you cook it to a higher temperature than medium, it will get very tough and chewy. Cooked simply like this, you can enjoy it on its own or on top of a salad or tacos; for something different, flavor it with your favorite marinade. Be sure to slice it on the thinner side for the best texture.

Prep: 5 minutes ■ Cook: 10 minutes ■ Serves: 4

1½ pounds flank steak
Fine sea salt and freshly ground black pepper
1 tablespoon avocado oil
2 cloves garlic, peeled and crashed with the side
  of a chef's knife

1. Allow the steak to sit at room temperature for at least 30 and up to 60 minutes before cooking. Thoroughly pat the steak dry. Cut the steak in half or thirds if needed to fit into the skillet.
2. Warm a large cast-iron or heavy-bottom stainless-steel skillet over medium-high heat until hot. Just before cooking, season the steak all over generously with salt and lightly with pepper. Swirl the oil in the skillet and add the steak. Let it cook undisturbed until the bottom is seared in spots, 3 to 4 minutes. Flip the steak. Add the garlic to the skillet. Using a silicone brush, brush the garlicky oil over the top of the steak several times.

3. Continue to cook, flipping once more and spooning more garlicky oil over the steak, until an instant-read thermometer inserted into the thickest part reads 130°F for medium-rare, 4 to 5 minutes longer, depending on the thickness of the steak. Transfer to a cutting board, tent with foil, and let rest for 5 to 10 minutes. Slice the steak thinly against the grain, and serve.

Per serving: 284 calories, 37 g protein, 0 g carbs, 14 g fat, 0 g fiber

Note: If your steak has a thick end and a thinner end, cut it so those pieces are separated. Cook each to 130°F (the thinner piece will cook faster). Be sure to cut against the grain. The grain is the direction the muscle fibers line up. With flank, it's really easy to see the grain, and it mostly runs in the same direction (with some cuts, such as rib eye, the grain can run in a few different directions in one steak, so you have to cut it into pieces just to slice it). Use your fingers to gently pull the meat apart so you can see the grain. Slice across it, perpendicularly. This shortens the grain, leaving you more tender meat that's easier to chew.

HERBED BEEF TENDERLOIN

If you're looking for a showstopping roast for a special occasion—or you're just feeling splurgy—this one's for you. Beef tenderloin (where filet mignon comes from) is the most tender cut of beef. It's also deceptively simple to cook, and, given its cylindrical shape and no bones, it's easy to carve as well. Though it's a lean cut, it's so flavorful and luscious. We use the reverse-sear method, where you cook it low and slow until just below medium-rare, then sear it in a hot skillet—a foolproof method for perfect results every time. The *Wild Mushroom Sauce* (page 346) goes beautifully with it.

Prep: 15 minutes ▪ Marinate: 1 hour ▪ Cook: 1 hour ▪ Serves: 8

2 pounds beef tenderloin, patted dry
1 tablespoon plus 2 teaspoons avocado oil
2 teaspoons chopped fresh rosemary
1 teaspoon chopped fresh thyme
2 cloves garlic, grated on a Microplane
Fine sea salt and freshly ground black pepper

1. Rub the meat all over with the 2 teaspoons oil, then rub with the rosemary, thyme, and garlic. Cover and refrigerate for at least 1 hour or up to overnight. Let the meat stand at room temperature for 30 to 60 minutes before cooking.

2. Preheat the oven to 300°F; line a rimmed baking sheet with parchment paper and place a wire cooling rack on top. Season the meat generously with salt and pepper. Using kitchen twine, tie the beef at 1-inch intervals. Place the meat on the baking sheet and bake until an instant-read thermometer inserted into the thickest part reads 125°F, 45 to 55 minutes, turning over halfway through.

3. Preheat a large cast-iron skillet over high heat. When it's hot, add the 1 tablespoon oil and swirl to coat the bottom of the

skillet. Add the beef tenderloin and cook, turning with tongs, until it's seared all over, 2 to 3 minutes. Transfer the beef to a cutting board, loosely tent with foil, and let it rest for 10 to 15 minutes.

4. Cut off the twine, slice the roast, and serve, or let it cool completely, wrap it, and refrigerate it to serve cold.

Per serving: 258 calories, 35 g protein, 0 g carbs, 13 g fat, 0 g fiber

UPGRADED GROUND BEEF
(BURGER SALAD) ("SPAGHETTI" WITH MEAT SAUCE)

Shredding just a bit of liver into ground beef is a convenient way to infuse it with good nutrition. You don't taste the liver, just a richer, more savory version of the ground beef you already love. Grating the liver while frozen is far easier than mincing it; it thaws quickly, so it combines easily into the meat, and you can keep any unused portion of the liver in the freezer for next time, so none of it goes to waste. Use this mixture for burgers, in your favorite meat loaf or meatball recipe, or cooked in a skillet and added to the *Spicy Tomato Sauce* (page 345) in this book for a delicious, supercharged meat sauce.

Prep: 10 minutes ■ Serves: 4

2 ounces beef liver, frozen
1 pound 6 ounces lean ground beef

Using the large holes of a box grater, shred the liver into a large bowl. Add the ground beef and, using your hands, gently but thoroughly combine the liver and beef. Cook as desired.

Per serving: 361 calories, 46 g protein, 1 g carbs, 18 g fat, 0 g fiber

TACO STUFFED PEPPERS WITH CILANTRO-LIME CREMA
(TACO STUFFED PEPPERS)

Make your Taco Tuesday (or whenever) delicious and super-nutrient-rich with this crowd-pleasing dish. You won't miss the tortillas at all. A nondairy, cashew-based crema full of cilantro and lime really enlivens the stuffed peppers and makes the dish feel special. You can make the filling and assemble the peppers, then cover and refrigerate and bake later, if you like. Leftover crema is fantastic drizzled on *Poached Chicken Breast* (page 312) or *Roasted Shrimp* (page 318).

Prep: 25 minutes ■ Stand: 4 hours ■ Cook: 50 minutes ■ Serves: 4

Crema:
> *1 cup raw cashews*
> *¾ cup cilantro leaves*
> *Zest of 1 lime plus 3 tablespoons lime juice*
> *Fine sea salt and freshly ground black pepper*

Peppers:
> *1 tablespoon avocado oil plus more for greasing*
> *4 medium bell peppers (any color)*
> *5 scallions, white and light green parts chopped (about ½ cup)*
> *Fine sea salt*
> *3 cloves garlic, minced (about 1 tablespoon)*
> *1 tablespoon chili powder*
> *1 teaspoon ground cumin*
> *¼ teaspoon smoked paprika*
> *Freshly ground black pepper*
> *1 pound 95% lean ground beef*
> *2 cups cauliflower rice, thawed and drained if frozen*
> *1 can (14.5 ounces) fire-roasted tomatoes with chilies, drained*
> *Taco toppings, such as pickled onion, avocado, radishes, salsa, or sliced ripe olives (optional)*

1. Make the crema: Cover the cashews with cool water. Cover and refrigerate for at least 4 hours or up to overnight. Drain and rinse the cashews; transfer to a high-speed blender or food processor. Add the cilantro, lime zest and juice, and ½ cup water; blend. Add more water as needed to reach sauce consistency. Taste and season with salt and black pepper. (Yield: 1½ cups. You can make crema up to 1 day ahead; cover and refrigerate.)

2. Make the peppers: Preheat the oven to 350°F. Lightly grease a 13 x 9-inch baking dish. Cut a bell pepper in half lengthwise, cutting through the stem. Remove the seeds and membranes; place the bell pepper halves cut sides up in a baking dish. Repeat with the remaining bell peppers. Warm the 1 tablespoon oil in a large skillet over medium heat. Add the scallions, sprinkle with salt, and cook, stirring occasionally, until tender, about 2 minutes. Add the garlic; sauté until fragrant, 1 minute. Add the chili powder, cumin, paprika, and a few turns of black pepper; sauté for 1 minute. Add the beef, season with salt, and cook, breaking up the meat, until nearly cooked through, 3 to 4 minutes. Add the cauliflower rice; sauté until warmed through, 2 minutes for thawed, 4 minutes for fresh. Stir in the tomatoes; remove from the heat. Taste and season with salt and black pepper. (Yield: about 6 cups.)

3. Spoon the beef mixture into the bell peppers, dividing evenly. Cover with foil and bake until the peppers are tender, 35 to 40 minutes. Be careful when uncovering the baking dish; escaping steam can burn. Let cool slightly. Drizzle each with 1 tablespoon crema, top with any desired taco toppings, and serve.

Per serving: 328 calories, 36 g protein, 17 g carbs, 13 g fat, 5 g fiber

Note: If you can't find canned tomatoes with chilies, seed and dice a fresh jalapeño and cook along with the scallions.

HERBED BURGER

(BURGER + EGGS) (BURGER + RICE)

Herbs elevate simple burgers into something special. This is also a perfect recipe to use the *Upgraded Ground Beef* (page 308), especially if you're cooking for someone who's really resistant to organ meats. The herbs thoroughly hide the richness of the liver. Enjoy these burgers with a lettuce wrap or on top of a salad.

Prep: 20 minutes ■ Cook: 1 hour ■ Serves: 4

1⅓ pounds 95% lean ground beef
¼ cup chopped fresh flat-leaf parsley
3 tablespoons chopped fresh basil
1½ teaspoons dried oregano
1½ teaspoons fine sea salt
½ teaspoon freshly ground black pepper
Avocado oil
Chopped romaine or other lettuce for serving, optional

1. In a large bowl, combine the beef, parsley, basil, oregano, salt, and pepper; mix gently but thoroughly with your hands to distribute the herbs. Divide into four portions; form into patties (*hint:* press the meat between two yogurt container lids to form patties without overworking the meat).
2. Warm a large skillet over medium-high heat; pour in the oil. Cook the burgers to the desired doneness, 2 to 4 minutes per side for medium-rare (an instant-read thermometer inserted into a burger should read 130°F). Serve the burgers on top of the lettuce, if desired.

Per serving: 267 calories, 42 g protein, 1 g carbs, 10 g fat, 0 g fiber

POACHED CHICKEN BREAST

Poaching is a moist-heat cooking method where you submerge food in a liquid with little or no fat and cook it gently. It's convenient because it's mostly hands-off, and with chicken, you're left with lightly flavored meat that you can then use in many different applications. Chop it and fold it into chicken salad, shred and add to soup, or toss with no-sugar barbecue sauce or hot sauce and enjoy with vegetables for a quick protein-rich meal. Make a batch on Sunday and use it for up to four days.

Prep: 10 minutes ■ Cook: 25 minutes ■ Serves: 4

1½ pounds boneless, skinless chicken breasts
3 cups chicken bone broth
Filtered water
½ teaspoon fine sea salt
2 large cloves garlic, or 3 small, peeled and crushed
with the side of a chef's knife
¼ teaspoon whole black peppercorns
3 sprigs fresh thyme

1. Pat the chicken dry and place in a wide deep skillet. Pour the broth over it, then add enough water until the chicken is submerged and stir in the salt. Add the garlic, peppercorns, and thyme; tuck into the liquid around the chicken.

2. Turn the heat to medium, and bring to a simmer (an instant-read thermometer inserted in the water should read between 170° and 180°F). Reduce the heat to low, gently turn the chicken breasts over, cover the skillet, and cook undisturbed for 10 minutes.

3. Place an instant-read thermometer into the thickest part of the chicken; it should read 165°F. If it isn't there yet, re-cover the skillet and cook 2 minutes longer, then check again. When the chicken has reached 165°F, remove the skillet from the heat, cover, and let stand for 5 minutes. Remove the chicken from the poaching liquid, and slice or shred. Alternatively, let the chicken cool, cover, and refrigerate to use later.

Per serving: 210 calories, 40 g protein, 0 g carbs, 5 g fat, 0 g fiber

Notes: If the chicken is much thicker on one side, before poaching, place it between two sheets of parchment, and lightly pound the thicker side with a rolling pin or wine bottle until the sides are closer to even.

It will take a little while for the liquid to reach 170°F; this is what you want. Resist the urge to crank the heat to make it hit the temperature faster. The low-and-slow cooking will yield you tender, moist chicken; going too fast and hot will make the chicken dry and rubbery.

This is a very neutral poaching liquid, so you can use the chicken in a variety of ways. Feel free to flavor the liquid if you know the chicken is going into a particular dish; for example, omit the thyme and add more garlic and several pieces of sliced ginger for an Asian-inspired dish, or add garlic and sliced jalapeños for a Mexican dish.

You can strain the poaching liquid and use it as a base for soup, a sauce or gravy, or the liquid to cook rice.

CRISP ROASTED CHICKEN THIGHS

Five minutes of prep and mostly hands-off cooking—just what you want for a meal on busy weeknights. Plus, though the white meat gets all the glory, dark meat has its advantages: Along with great flavor, chicken thighs have more iron, zinc, and B vitamins than breasts. Buying dark meat and choosing bone-in, skin-on is economical too.

Prep: 5 minutes ■ Cook: 28 minutes ■ Serves: 4

2 teaspoons garlic powder
¾ teaspoon smoked paprika
2 pounds bone-in, skin-on chicken thighs (4 to 8,
*   depending on size), patted dry*
Fine sea salt and freshly ground black pepper
1 tablespoon avocado oil

1. Preheat the oven to 425°F. Place a large cast-iron skillet in the oven as it preheats. In a small bowl, mix the garlic powder and paprika.
2. Season the chicken generously with salt and pepper. Rub all over with the garlic mixture. When the oven reaches temperature, carefully remove the skillet and place over medium heat. Swirl the oil in the skillet and add the chicken, skin side down. Cover with a splatter guard or loosely cover with foil and cook until the skin is golden brown and crisp and releases easily from the skillet, 6 to 8 minutes.
3. Flip the chicken thighs over, transfer the skillet back to the oven, and cook until the chicken is cooked through (an instant-read thermometer inserted into the thickest part, away from the bone, should read 165°F), 15 to 20 minutes. Serve hot.

Per serving: 411 calories, 29 g protein, 5 g carbs, 32 g fat, 1 g fiber

Note: You can make these chicken thighs in an air fryer, if you like. Preheat the fryer to 400°F. Mist the basket with olive or

*avocado oil cooking spray. Place the spice-rubbed chicken in the
fryer skin side down; cook until golden and crisp, 8 to 10 minutes. Flip the chicken and air fry until the internal temperature
reaches 165°F, 8 to 12 minutes longer (depending on how large
they are).*

GREEN GODDESS COBB SALAD

If you're into meal prepping, this is the perfect salad for you. You can
make nearly everything in advance and then just throw it all together
when it's time to eat. Feel free to change up the ingredients for the
salad based on what you have on hand: leftover cooked green beans
or broccoli could make up a row, you could swap shrimp for chicken,
you could start with a different kind of lettuce—you can make your
Cobb salad different every time. Green goddess dressing is a labor of
love (picking all those herbs!) but so worth it—though, of course, you
can grab a high-quality bottled version if you're short on time.

Prep: 30 minutes ■ Cook: 30 minutes ■ Serves: 4

Dressing:

2 tablespoons extra-virgin olive oil

1 clove garlic, minced (about 1 teaspoon)

1 small ripe avocado

3 tablespoons snipped chives

2 tablespoons chopped fresh tarragon

¼ cup fresh parsley leaves

¼ cup chopped fresh basil

2 tablespoons lemon juice

2 tablespoons avocado oil mayonnaise

2 teaspoons coconut aminos

Fine sea salt and freshly ground black pepper

Salad:

    6 cups chopped romaine lettuce

    2 slices bacon, cooked until crisp, crumbled

    2 large eggs, hard-cooked to desired doneness, quartered

    12 ounces boneless, skinless chicken breast, cooked and cut
        into cubes (see Poached Chicken Breast, *page 312)*

    2 cups halved cherry tomatoes

    3 tablespoons sliced ripe black olives

1. Make the dressing: Combine the oil and garlic in a small unheated skillet. Place over low heat and cook until the mixture sizzles, about 30 seconds, then transfer to a cup to cool. Combine the avocado, chives, tarragon, parsley, basil, lemon juice, mayonnaise, and coconut aminos in a high-speed blender or small food processor. Add the cooled garlic mixture and process until smooth. Thin with water if needed to reach the desired consistency. Taste and season with salt and pepper. (Yield: 1¼ cups. You can make the dressing up to two days ahead; cover and refrigerate.)

2. Make the salad: Toss the lettuce with ¼ cup dressing. (Toss again with more dressing if you like.) Divide among four bowls. Make rows on top of the lettuce with the bacon, eggs, chicken, tomatoes, and olives, dividing the ingredients evenly. Drizzle with more dressing, if desired, and serve.

Per serving: 283 calories, 33 g protein, 8 g carbs, 13 g fat, 4 g fiber

GARLIC ROSEMARY ROAST PORK TENDERLOIN
(PORK + SWEET POTATOES) (PORK LOIN + VEG)

Brining pork tenderloin gives it lots of flavor and a really nice texture. Don't brine longer than four hours, or it can get mushy. There's no need to salt the meat again; the brine takes care of that.

Prep: 15 minutes ■ Brine: 1 to 4 hours ■ Cook: 20 minutes ■ Serves: 4

6 tablespoons kosher salt
2 dried bay leaves
1¼ pounds pork tenderloin, trimmed of excess fat
    and silver skin and patted dry
1 teaspoon lemon zest
1 teaspoon minced fresh rosemary
2 cloves garlic, minced (about 2 teaspoons)
1 tablespoon plus ½ teaspoon avocado oil
⅛ teaspoon freshly ground black pepper

1. In a large bowl, combine the salt with 2 cups water; stir to dissolve the salt. Stir in 2 cups cool water and the bay leaves. Add the pork; push to submerge in the brine. Cover and refrigerate for at least 1 hour and up to 4 hours.

2. Preheat the oven to 400°F; place a large cast-iron skillet in the oven as it preheats. Place the zest, rosemary, garlic, the ½ teaspoon oil, and the pepper on a cutting board. Chop together with a sharp chef's knife, turning the mixture over and continuing to chop until the mixture is very well combined and nearly a paste consistency. Remove the pork from the brine; pat dry thoroughly.

3. Carefully remove the hot skillet from the oven; place over medium-high heat and add the 1 tablespoon oil. Cook the pork, turning with tongs, until seared, 2 to 3 minutes per side.

Remove from the heat and top the pork with the rub. Transfer the skillet to the oven and roast until an instant-read thermometer inserted into the thickest part reads 135° to 140°F, 14 to 17 minutes. Transfer to a cutting board, cover with foil, and let rest for 10 minutes (internal temperature will continue to rise as the meat rests). Cut into slices and serve.

Per serving: 192 calories, 30 g protein, 1 g carbs, 7 g fat, 0 g fiber

ROASTED SHRIMP
(SHRIMP STIR-FRY)

Say goodbye to rubbery, overcooked shrimp forever. Roasting them for just a few minutes will yield you tender, just-crisped shrimp every time. Enjoy them hot, or let them cool, cover, and refrigerate for the best shrimp cocktail. Along with being perfectly tasty, shrimp are a great source of minerals such as selenium, iodine, zinc, and magnesium.

Prep: 5 minutes ■ Cook: 10 minutes ■ Serves: 4

2 pounds medium shrimp, peeled and deveined
1½ tablespoons olive oil or avocado oil
Fine sea salt and freshly ground black pepper

1. Preheat the oven to 400°F. Line two rimmed baking sheets with parchment paper.
2. Thoroughly pat the shrimp dry. Place them in a bowl, add the oil, and season with salt and pepper. Spread the shrimp in a single layer on the baking sheets and roast until they're just cooked through (they'll turn pink and curl slightly into a C shape), 8 to 10 minutes. Serve hot, or let cool, place in a container, cover, and refrigerate to serve cold.

Per serving: 205 calories, 30 g protein, 4 g carbs, 9 g fat, 0 g fiber

POACHED SALMON
(SALMON + SALAD + RICE) (SALMON + BEET SALAD)

Poached salmon is elegant and versatile, easy to make for a crowd or you can poach one serving just for yourself. Serve it for brunch or dinner, have it hot or cold, enjoy it with a sauce (*Yogurt-Dill Sauce* on page 344 and *Cilantro Pesto* on page 341 are both good options). Poaching is also a great option if you find cooking fish intimidating—it's simple to do and won't make your kitchen smell fishy (we promise).

Prep: 10 minutes ■ Cook: 15 minutes ■ Serves: 4

1 lemon, thinly sliced
½ teaspoon whole black peppercorns
2 cups dry white wine
1 dried bay leaf
1½ pounds wild-caught salmon, skin removed and cut into 4 pieces
1 tablespoon extra-virgin olive oil
Fine sea salt

1. Place the lemon slices and peppercorns in a large skillet with high sides. Pour in the wine and 2 cups water; add the bay leaf. Bring to a boil over medium-high heat, then reduce to medium-low.
2. Thoroughly pat the salmon dry. Drizzle with the oil and season all over with salt. Place an instant-read thermometer into the poaching liquid; it should read between 170° and 180°F. Place the salmon in the skillet on top of the lemon slices. Add more hot water if needed to just cover the salmon.
3. Cover and poach until the salmon is just cooked through (press the thickest part with a fork; it should flake easily), 8 to 12 minutes, depending on the thickness. Season with additional salt. Serve the salmon warm, or let cool, cover, and refrigerate to serve cold.

Per serving: 284 calories, 37 g protein, 0 g carbs, 14 g fat, 0 g fiber

ROASTED COD WITH LEMON-CAPER SAUCE

This is a really quick recipe that works well for a weeknight but is dressed-up enough to make for dinner guests. The sauce is more like a relish than a traditional sauce; if you'd like it thinner, add about ¼ cup white wine and reduce it by half before adding the cold butter.

Prep: 10 minutes ■ Cook: 15 minutes ■ Serves: 4

1½ pounds cod
2 tablespoons extra-virgin olive oil
Fine sea salt and freshly ground black pepper
2 tablespoons unsalted butter
1 small shallot, minced (about ¼ cup)
1 clove garlic, minced (about 1 teaspoon)
1 tablespoon drained capers, coarsely chopped
1 teaspoon lemon zest
2 tablespoons lemon juice
1 tablespoon chopped fresh flat-leaf parsley

1. Preheat the oven to 400°F; line a large baking sheet with parchment paper. Thoroughly pat the fish dry with paper towels. Rub all over with 1 tablespoon of the oil; season with salt and pepper. Roast the fish until it's cooked through and flakes easily with a fork, 12 to 15 minutes, depending on the thickness.

2. Meanwhile, make the sauce: Melt 1 tablespoon of the butter with the remaining 1 tablespoon oil in a small skillet over medium heat. (Put the other 1 tablespoon butter back in the fridge.) Add the shallot and a pinch of salt; cook, stirring occasionally, until the shallot is tender, 2 to 3 minutes. Add the garlic and capers; sauté until the garlic and capers are fragrant, about 1 minute. Whisk in the lemon zest and juice. Remove from the heat, and add the remaining 1 tablespoon butter a

piece at a time until the sauce is well incorporated. Whisk in the parsley, then taste and season with salt and pepper.

3. Divide the fish among four plates, spoon the sauce over it, and serve.

Per serving: 251 calories, 30 g protein, 2 g carbs, 14 g fat, 1 g fiber

SCRAMBLED EGGS

There are a zillion ways to make eggs, but these three are the ones we turn to the most. Paying attention to the temperature and other subtleties in each method will yield you the best results—nice, fluffy scrambled eggs instead of a dry, rubbery mess, for example. One large egg has 6 grams of protein, so even with three on your plate, it's not quite enough to reach your per-meal goal. Have a couple of slices of smoked salmon, a burger patty, some leftover chicken, or another protein with your eggs to round out the plate.

Serves: 1

3 large eggs
1 teaspoon ghee, avocado oil, or olive oil
Fine sea salt

In a medium bowl, whisk the eggs until well combined. Melt the ghee (or warm the oil) in a medium nonstick skillet over medium-low heat. Pour in the eggs, season with salt, and cook, stirring slowly but constantly with a silicone spatula. You want to keep the eggs from sticking to the skillet but allow the mixture to form large, fluffy curds. Cook until your desired level of doneness, 1 to 3 minutes. Serve hot.

Per serving: 247 calories, 18 g protein, 0 g carbs, 19 g fat, 0 g fiber

Notes: Medium-low is the temperature you need to get fluffy eggs. Low temp will get you very creamy eggs, which is nice, but it takes much longer. Higher heat will cause unevenly cooked, dried-out scrambled eggs.

Season your eggs however you like. A dash of sea salt is all you need, but feel free to add black pepper, fresh or dried herbs, or one of my favorites, Pluck seasoning, a mix of spices and freeze-dried organ meats. You don't taste the organs, just a really nice, savory seasoning.

FRIED EGGS
Serves: 1

1 tablespoon ghee
2 to 3 large eggs
Fine sea salt

Melt the ghee in a medium nonstick skillet over medium heat. Crack the eggs carefully into the skillet (or into a cup, then pour into the skillet); season with salt. Cook, gently tilting the skillet, spooning up the ghee and pouring it over the whites, until the whites are firm and the yolks are still runny, about 3 minutes. Serve hot.

Per serving (3 large eggs): 292 calories, 18 g protein, 3 g carbs, 25 g fat, 0 g fiber

Notes: Ghee tastes especially good here, but any high-heat fat will do. Avocado oil also works nicely.

If you prefer the yolks more cooked, you can baste them with the fat as you do with the whites, or flip them over and cook for 1 to 2 minutes.

STEAMED EGGS
(SHAKE + EGGS) (SALMON + SALAD + RICE)
Serves: 6

6 large eggs

Bring 1 inch of water to a boil in a large saucepan over medium-high heat. Place a steamer basket in the water. Add the eggs, cover the pan tightly, and allow the eggs to steam to the desired doneness, 8 to 9 minutes for jammy yolks, 10 to 11 minutes for firmer but still soft yolks, or 12 to 13 minutes for firm yolks. Just before the eggs are done, fill a bowl with ice water. When the eggs are done, use a slotted spoon to transfer them from the pan into the ice bath. Let cool, then peel and serve, or leave the shells on and refrigerate to use later.

Per serving (1 large egg): 70 calories, 6 g protein, 0 g carbs, 5 g fat, 0 g fiber

Note: Steaming eggs is the best way to hard-cook them, much better than submerging them in boiling water. For one thing, they're much easier to peel—no more stripping away a quarter-inch of egg white or scraping off a centimeter of peel at a time. Steaming is also a gentler cooking method, so you don't end up with that gross green ring around the yolks. Once you try steaming, you'll never go back to boiling.

"PERFECT" PORK CHOP
(PORK CHOP + VEGETABLES)

A bone-in pork chop is so satisfying; there's something primal about a generous chop cooked on the bone. Don't skip the brining step; it infuses the chops with flavor and makes them really tender. Even a 30-minute brine makes a difference.

Prep: 10 minutes ▪ **Brine: 30 minutes** ▪ **Cook: 12 minutes** ▪ **Serves: 4**

4 cups cold water
2 tablespoons fine sea salt
1 dried bay leaf
1 clove garlic, peeled and crushed with the side of a chef's knife
4 center-cut, bone-in pork chops (¾ to 1 inch thick)
1 tablespoon avocado oil
Freshly ground black pepper
Flaky sea salt, such as Maldon (optional)

1. In a saucepan, bring 1 cup of the water to a boil. Remove from the heat and stir in the salt until it dissolves. Add the bay leaf and garlic. Stir in the remaining 3 cups water. (If the brine is still warm, add a few ice cubes and let them melt before continuing.) Place the chops in a large shallow dish; pour the brine on top. Cover and refrigerate for at least 30 minutes or up to 8 hours. Remove the chops from the brine; pat dry thoroughly. Let the chops sit at room temperature for 30 minutes.

2. Preheat the oven to 400°F; place a large heavy-bottomed or cast-iron skillet in the oven as it preheats. Rub the chops all over with the oil; season with pepper. Carefully remove the hot skillet from the oven and place over medium-high heat. Add the chops to the skillet and cook undisturbed until seared on the bottom, 3 to 4 minutes. Flip and transfer the skillet back to the oven.

3. Cook the chops until an instant-read thermometer inserted into the thickest part of a chop, away from the bone, reads 145°F, 4 to 7 minutes, depending on the thickness. Transfer the chops to a cutting board, tent with foil, and let rest for 5 to 10 minutes before serving. Sprinkle lightly with flaky sea salt just before serving, if desired.

Per serving: 285 calories, 32 g protein, 0 g carbs, 17 g fat, 0 g fiber

Note: You can make a quick sauce with the drippings in the pan. Sauté a chopped shallot in the skillet, then pour in a tablespoon or two of white wine or vinegar and stir up the browned bits on the bottom of the skillet. When it has mostly evaporated, add ⅓ cup of broth and ½ to 1 teaspoon of Dijon mustard, and cook, whisking, until the sauce reduces and thickens. Taste and whisk in a little honey, and/or season with salt and pepper, if needed.

WALNUT-CRUSTED COD
(COD WITH BAKED POTATO)

Walnuts and a few pantry basics lend mild cod lots of flavor and texture. This dish is easy enough for a weeknight but dressed-up enough for dinner guests. If cod isn't available, you can swap in another firm white fish, such as haddock, hake, or pollock.

Prep: 15 minutes ■ Cook: 12 minutes ■ Serves: 4

½ cup chopped walnuts
1 teaspoon dried dill
½ teaspoon lemon zest
¼ teaspoon garlic powder
¼ teaspoon paprika
Fine sea salt and freshly ground black pepper

1 teaspoon avocado oil mayonnaise
2 teaspoons Dijon mustard
1½ pounds cod, cut into 4 portions (thawed if frozen)
1 tablespoon extra-virgin olive oil

1. Preheat the oven to 400°F. Line a rimmed baking sheet with parchment paper.
2. Place the walnuts, dill, lemon zest, garlic powder, paprika, and a pinch each of salt and pepper on a cutting board. Finely chop, turning the mixture over several times to make sure everything is incorporated. (Alternatively, if you have a small food processor, pulse the ingredients together until finely chopped and well combined.) In a cup, mix the mayonnaise and mustard.
3. Thoroughly pat the fish dry, season all over with salt and pepper, and place on the baking sheet. Spread a very thin layer of the mustard mixture over each piece of fish. Divide the walnut mixture among the fish pieces, pressing it to adhere. Drizzle the fish with the oil.
4. Bake until the fish is just cooked through (it should flake easily with a fork), 10 to 12 minutes. Serve hot.

Per serving: 277 calories, 33 g protein, 3 g carbs, 15 g fat, 1 g fiber

SIDES

GREEN BEANS AND SHALLOTS WITH ALMONDS
(STEAK + GREEN BEANS)

Simple green beans get dressed up with sliced almonds and shallots, though this dish is still on the table in less than 30 minutes. Thin green beans, often labeled *haricots verts* in the supermarket (though that just translates to "green beans" in French), are best for this dish. Cooking them quickly in boiling salted water—blanching—takes the raw edge off before you finish them quickly in a skillet.

Prep: 15 minutes ■ Cook: 10 minutes ■ Serves: 4

Fine sea salt
1 pound thin green beans (haricots verts), trimmed
1½ tablespoons ghee
3 tablespoons sliced almonds
3 small shallots, or 2 medium, chopped (about ¾ cup)
2 cloves garlic, minced (about 2 teaspoons)
1 tablespoon lemon juice
Freshly ground black pepper

1. Bring a pot of salted water to a boil. Add the green beans and cook until bright green and just crisp-tender, 2 to 3 minutes. Drain.
2. Melt 1 tablespoon of the ghee in a large skillet over medium heat. Add the almonds and cook, stirring, until lightly toasted, 1 to 2 minutes. Add the shallots and a pinch of salt; cook, stirring, until the shallots have softened, about 1 minute. Add the garlic; sauté until fragrant, about 1 minute.

3. Add the green beans to the skillet along with the remaining ½ tablespoon ghee and the lemon juice; season lightly with salt. Cook, tossing, until the green beans are coated and everything is well combined and hot. Taste and season with pepper and additional salt, if needed. Serve hot.

Per serving: 134 calories, 5 g protein, 15 g carbs, 8 g fat, 6 g fiber

ROASTED RADISHES AND RADISH GREENS

If you think you don't like radishes, but you haven't had them cooked, you're in for a treat. Roasting radishes eases their peppery bite and gives them a texture similar to thin-skinned waxy potatoes. The greens, which often come attached, are also delicious, with a slightly bitter edge that's softened with cooking and the addition of a splash of acid. We use cider vinegar, but you can swap in lemon if you prefer.

Prep: 25 minutes ■ Cook: 30 minutes ■ Serves: 2 to 4

3 bunches radishes with greens (about 30 radishes and
*   2 cups greens)*
1 tablespoon avocado oil
Fine sea salt and freshly ground black pepper
½ teaspoon garlic powder
1 teaspoon dried rosemary, lightly crushed with your fingers
1 teaspoon cider vinegar

1. Preheat the oven to 450°F. Place a large heavy-bottomed or cast-iron skillet in the oven as it preheats.
2. Use kitchen shears to snip the greens off the radishes. Trim and halve the radishes (or cut into quarters or sixths if large) and

place in a large bowl (reserve the greens). Drizzle the radishes with the oil; season generously with salt and pepper and sprinkle in the garlic powder and rosemary. Toss to coat the radishes with the oil and seasonings. Carefully remove the hot skillet from the oven and spread the radishes in a single layer in the skillet. Roast the radishes until they are very tender and caramelized in spots, 20 to 25 minutes, tossing halfway through.

3. While the radishes are roasting, fill a bowl with cold water and add the radish greens. Swish them around to remove any grit. Carefully lift the greens out of the water; thoroughly pat dry. (Alternatively, use a salad spinner to thoroughly wash and dry the greens.) Coarsely chop the greens.

4. Carefully remove the hot skillet from the oven and place it on the stove over medium heat. Add the greens, sprinkle with the vinegar and salt, and cook, stirring, until the greens have wilted, 1 to 2 minutes. Taste and season with additional salt and pepper, if needed. Serve hot. (Yield: about 3 cups.)

Per serving: 78 calories, 1 g protein, 4 g carbs, 7 g fat, 2 g fiber

Notes: This dish is tasty hot, at room temperature, or cold. Try it with the Cilantro Pesto *(page 341) or* Lemon-Herb Tahini Sauce *(page 342) drizzled on or topped with a small dollop of plain Greek yogurt. Toss any leftovers into a salad.*

If you buy radishes with the greens attached and you aren't going to cook them the same day, snip off the greens close to the tops of the radishes and store them separately. (Wash and dry the greens thoroughly, then wrap the greens in a slightly damp paper towel and store in a plastic bag in the fridge.) If the greens remain attached, they'll leach moisture out of the radishes. The same goes for beets and carrots.

STIR-FRIED VEGETABLES
(SHRIMP STIR-FRY)

Stir-frying is a high-heat cooking method that moves very fast, so make sure all of your ingredients are prepped and ready before you turn on the stove. Having everything chopped, diced, and otherwise prepped—a process chefs call *mise en place*—will save you from over-cooking anything. The best stir-fried vegetables are loaded with flavor, cooked nicely but still crisp-tender to the bite.

Prep: 25 minutes ■ Cook: 12 minutes ■ Serves: 4

3 tablespoons coconut aminos

1 teaspoon unseasoned rice vinegar

½ teaspoon arrowroot

2 tablespoons avocado oil

5 ounces sliced shiitake mushroom caps (about 3 cups)

Fine sea salt

6 scallions, white and light green parts sliced; slice and reserve
    the dark green parts for garnish (about 1 cup), optional

1 small red bell pepper, seeded and chopped (about ¾ cup)

1 bunch asparagus (about 1 pound), tough ends trimmed
    and sliced diagonally into 2-inch pieces (about 4 cups)

3 cloves garlic, minced (about 1 tablespoon)

1 tablespoon minced fresh ginger

2 teaspoons toasted sesame oil

Sriracha, optional

1. In a small bowl, combine the coconut aminos, rice vinegar, and arrowroot.

2. Warm 1 tablespoon of the avocado oil in a large skillet over medium-high heat. Add the mushrooms, season with salt, and cook, stirring occasionally, until they release their water

and begin to turn golden in spots, 5 to 7 minutes. Add the remaining 1 tablespoon avocado oil and the scallions, bell pepper, and asparagus; season with salt and cook, stirring, until just beginning to get tender, 2 to 3 minutes.

3. Stir in the garlic and ginger; sauté until fragrant, 30 seconds to 1 minute. Add the coconut aminos mixture; cook, stirring constantly, until the sauce thickens and coats the vegetables, about 1 minute. Remove from the heat, drizzle with the sesame oil and sriracha, if using, and serve. (Yield: about 5 cups.)

Per serving: 152 calories, 5 g protein, 15 g carbs, 10 g fat, 4 g fiber

BONE BROTH RICE
(SHRIMP STIR-FRY) (SALMON + BEET SALAD) (BURGER + RICE) (STEAK + VEG + RICE) (SALMON + SALAD + RICE)

Cooking rice in bone broth not only gives it some essential nutrients, but it also lends plain rice a rich, satisfying flavor. Enjoy it as a side dish on its own, or have it with the *Stir-Fried Vegetables* (page 330) and your protein of choice. Chicken bone broth is my favorite for rice, but beef or any other variety will work well.

Prep: 5 minutes ■ Cook: 23 minutes ■ Yield: about 4 cups

1 cup long grain white rice
1¾ cups chicken bone broth
1 tablespoon unsalted butter, optional
½ teaspoon fine sea salt

1. Place the rice in a fine-mesh sieve. Rinse with cold water, stirring the rice with your fingers, until the water that comes out the bottom is less cloudy. (If you can't see the water well enough to tell, place a bowl under the sieve and collect the water to see.)

2. Place the broth in a medium saucepan; add the butter, if using. Turn the heat to medium and bring the broth to just a boil. Stir in the rice and salt. Bring the water back to a simmer, reduce the heat to low (as low as it will go), cover the pot, and cook undisturbed until the broth has been absorbed and the rice is tender, 18 to 22 minutes. To check that all of the liquid has been absorbed, do not stir. Gently tip the pot and check for excess liquid; if you see any, cover the pot and continue to cook on low in 2-minute intervals until the liquid has been absorbed. Do not stir.

3. Once all the broth has been absorbed, remove the pot from the heat, cover, and let stand undisturbed for 5 minutes. Fluff the rice with a fork, and serve, or transfer to a bowl, let cool, cover, and refrigerate to use later.

Per serving (½ cup cooked): 110 calories, 4 g protein, 22 g carbs, 0 g fat, 0 g fiber

AIR-FRIED ARTICHOKE HEARTS

Artichokes—part of the thistle family—can be a bit fussy to prepare, which is why jarred or canned artichoke hearts are so popular. Luckily, the hearts are loaded with antioxidants, so you can eat them on their own and not worry about missing out on the nutrition in the rest of the plant. Air-frying them makes them pleasingly crisp and a fun appetizer. Try dipping them in *Yogurt-Dill Sauce* (page 344).

Prep: 10 minutes ■ Cook: 9 minutes ■ Serves: 2 to 4

1 can (14.1 ounces) quartered artichoke hearts, drained
2 teaspoons extra-virgin olive oil
1 teaspoon Italian seasoning

Pinch of crushed red pepper flakes, optional
Fine sea salt and freshly ground black pepper
Olive or avocado oil cooking spray

1. Preheat an air fryer to 400°F. Thoroughly pat the artichoke hearts dry. Place them in a bowl, add the oil, Italian seasoning, and red pepper flakes, if using, and toss to coat. Season lightly with salt and black pepper.

2. Mist the air fryer basket with cooking spray. Spread the artichoke hearts in a single layer in the basket and cook until beginning to turn crisp and golden in spots, about 4 minutes. Flip the artichoke hearts, and cook until crisper and more golden all over, 3 to 5 minutes longer. Serve hot.

Per serving: 101 calories, 3 g protein, 14 g carbs, 5 g fat, 7 g fiber

Notes: If quartered artichoke hearts aren't readily available, buy whole or halved, and cut into quarters.

This timing will give you artichoke hearts that are crisp on the edges and outsides, tender inside. Turn them again and cook for an additional 3 to 6 minutes to get them crisper (remove them as they brown to avoid burning).

You can double or triple the recipe easily to feed a crowd, but you'll need to cook in batches to get that golden color and crispness. Place a cooling rack on top of a baking sheet and preheat the oven to 200°F. As each batch finishes cooking, spread the cooked artichoke hearts on the rack in the oven to keep them warm while the remaining batches cook.

These lose their crispness pretty quickly after coming out of the fryer, so plan to cook them just before eating them.

SHREDDED BEET AND CARROT SALAD
WITH CUMIN-ORANGE VINAIGRETTE
(TUNA + BEET SALAD) (SALMON + BEET SALAD)
(SALMON + SALAD + RICE)

Beets are usually steamed or roasted, but they actually work beautifully raw. Their earthiness pairs nicely with sweet carrots, and an easy vinaigrette with orange juice and cumin lends complexity. We used a single chopped date in place of the raisins that are traditional in carrot salad; just a hint of chewy sweetness is all you really need, and the whole thing comes together with salty, crunchy pistachios on top. Serve this with grilled meat, fish, or really any protein you like. Watch out when prepping; beets will stain your light-colored clothes.

Prep: 20 minutes ■ Serves: 4

½ teaspoon Dijon mustard
½ teaspoon grated orange zest
2 tablespoons orange juice
1 tablespoon apple cider vinegar
½ teaspoon raw honey
¼ teaspoon ground cumin
Pinch of cayenne, optional
2 tablespoons extra-virgin olive oil
Fine sea salt and freshly ground black pepper
2 small beets, or 1 large, peeled and shredded (about 2 cups)
3 medium carrots, shredded (about 2 cups)
1 pitted dried date, minced
2 tablespoons finely chopped roasted, salted pistachios

1. Make the dressing: In a medium bowl, whisk together the mustard, orange zest and juice, vinegar, honey, cumin, and cayenne, if using. While whisking, drizzle in the oil. Continue

whisking until well mixed. Taste and season with salt and black pepper. (Yield: ¼ cup.)

3. Place the shredded beets in a fine-meshed sieve; gently rinse with cold water. Pat dry thoroughly and place in a medium bowl. Add the carrots and date; gently toss. Add 3 tablespoons of the dressing and toss again. (Add the remaining 1 tablespoon dressing if the salad seems dry.) Taste and season with salt and black pepper. Let the salad stand at room temperature for at least 20 minutes to allow the vegetables to become more tender and the flavors to develop. (Yield: about 3 cups.)

2. Toss the salad again, sprinkle with the pistachios, and serve.

Per serving: 121 calories, 2 g protein, 12 g carbs, 8 g fat, 3 g fiber

Notes: Use a food processor with a shredding blade for the carrots and beets, if you have one. A box grater will work, but with the beets it can get very messy.

If the salad sits for a while, liquid will collect at the bottom. Spoon the salad out of the liquid (or pull out with tongs) to serve.

TANGY COLESLAW
(PORK + SWEET POTATOES)

Coleslaw is always a crowd-pleaser. Using a packaged coleslaw mix, with shredded cabbage and carrot, makes tossing this together fast and easy. (*Pro tip:* You can also sauté coleslaw mix to make a fast egg-roll bowl.) Letting the scallion sit in the vinegar for a few minutes softens its bite so it doesn't overpower the flavors in the rest of the bowl.

Prep: 20 minutes ■ Serves: 6

*1 scallion, white and light green parts thinly sliced
    on a diagonal (about 2 tablespoons)*
3 tablespoons apple cider vinegar
*1 bag (14 ounces) coleslaw mix (about 7 cups shredded
    cabbage and carrots)*
1 small red bell pepper, seeded and thinly sliced (about 1 cup)
1 tablespoon Dijon mustard
2 teaspoons coconut aminos
2 teaspoons raw honey
1 teaspoon ground celery seed
3 tablespoons extra-virgin olive oil
Fine sea salt and freshly ground black pepper

1. In a small cup, combine the scallion and vinegar; let stand for at least 15 minutes.
2. In a large bowl, combine the coleslaw mix and bell pepper. In a small bowl, whisk together the mustard, coconut aminos, honey, and celery seed. Spoon the scallion out of the vinegar, and add it to the bowl with the coleslaw mix, then whisk the vinegar into the mustard mixture. Whisking constantly, whisk in the oil until well mixed and emulsified. Taste and season with salt and black pepper.

3. Add the vinegar mixture to the coleslaw mixture and use tongs to toss well. Taste and season with more salt and pepper, if needed. Serve. (Yield: about 5½ cups.)

Per serving: 97 calories; 1 g protein, 7 g carbs, 7 g fat, 2 g fiber

Note: Between the acid in the vinegar and the salt, the cabbage will relax pretty quickly once the coleslaw mix is combined with the dressing. If you want to make this in advance but have it remain crisp when serving, make the vegetable mix and the dressing, cover separately, and toss together just before serving.

MASHED PURPLE SWEET POTATOES WITH SESAME
(PORK + SWEET POTATOES)

Talk about a dramatic dish: the bright color of these sweet potatoes not only looks amazing, but it also indicates that this dish is loaded with anthocyanin pigments, immune-boosting and inflammation-fighting antioxidants. Roasting them instead of boiling takes longer, but the flavor is so much richer, and this method preserves more of that beautiful color. The tahini and sesame oil give the dish richness and depth.

Prep: 15 minutes ■ Cook: 1 hour 30 minutes ■ Serves: 8

2 pounds purple sweet potatoes (such as Frieda's Stokes),
    scrubbed and dried
1 cup milk of choice (I used almond)
¼ cup tahini
1 teaspoon ground ginger
2 teaspoons coconut aminos
1 teaspoon toasted sesame oil
Fine sea salt
Sesame seeds for garnish, optional

1. Preheat the oven to 400°F. Wrap the potatoes in a layer of parchment paper, covered by a sheet of foil. Place on a large rimmed baking sheet and bake until the potatoes are very fragrant and tender (a paring knife inserted into the thickest part should go in easily), 1 hour to 1 hour 30 minutes.
2. In a medium saucepan, combine the milk, tahini, and ginger; bring to a simmer over medium-low heat, stirring to combine. Remove from the heat.
3. Carefully unwrap the potatoes, trim off the edges, and halve lengthwise. Scoop the flesh out of the skins and add it to the saucepan, along with the coconut aminos and oil. Use a potato masher, fork, or immersion blender to mash the potatoes and combine all the ingredients. Taste and season with salt. Transfer to a bowl, sprinkle with sesame seeds, if desired, and serve. (Yield: about 4 cups.)

Per serving (½ cup): 211 calories, 4 g protein, 37 g carbs, 5 g fat, 5 g fiber

BRAISED RADICCHIO AND ENDIVE
(PORK LOIN + VEG) (STEAK + VEG + RICE)

We associate braising with tougher cuts of meat, but cooking vegetables low and slow in a bit of liquid gives them great flavor. Both radicchio and endive are bitter greens, and the combination of the braise, a touch of honey, and a little acid from the lemon softens that edge, so you end up with kind of a dressed-up version of sweet and sour. Use all endive or all radicchio instead of the combination, if you prefer.

Prep: 10 minutes ■ Cook: 50 minutes ■ Serves: 4

1 tablespoon ghee
3 heads endive, trimmed, halved lengthwise, and brown
    or damaged outer leaves removed

3 small heads radicchio, trimmed, halved lengthwise,
*   and brown or damaged outer leaves removed*
2 tablespoons lemon juice
1 teaspoon raw honey
⅓ cup chicken bone broth
Fine sea salt

1. Have ready a piece of parchment paper cut to fit inside a large ovenproof skillet with a cover or a Dutch oven. Preheat the oven to 375°F.

2. Melt the ghee in the skillet over medium heat. Add the endive and radicchio, cut sides down. Sprinkle with the lemon juice and drizzle with the honey, then carefully pour in the broth (pour it into the sides of the skillet, not over the vegetables). Season the vegetables with salt. Bring to a simmer.

3. Place the parchment gently over the vegetables, then cover the skillet. Transfer the skillet to the oven and braise until the vegetables are very tender and the bottoms are golden, 30 to 40 minutes.

4. Carefully transfer the skillet back to the stove and place it over medium heat. Uncover and remove the parchment. Turn the vegetables over with tongs and continue to cook until the vegetables are golden in spots all over and the liquid has evaporated, 5 to 10 minutes longer, turning once or twice more. Taste and season with additional salt, if needed. Serve hot, or let cool, cover, and refrigerate to serve cold.

Per serving: 147 calories, 8 g protein, 23 g carbs, 5 g fat, 14 g fiber

ROASTED BRUSSELS SPROUTS, CARROTS, AND ONIONS
(PORK CHOP + VEGETABLES)

Roasting vegetables makes them tender and brings out their sweetness, thanks to caramelization. This is a very forgiving recipe; feel free to swap other vegetables depending on what's available and your taste. Try parsnips or winter squash instead of the carrots, broccoli or cauliflower instead of the Brussels sprouts, any other kind of onion instead of yellow (be sure to cut the onions into thick slices so they don't overbrown while the other vegetables cook). Also, use thyme instead of rosemary, or use both.

Prep: 20 minutes ■ Cook: 45 minutes ■ Serves: 4

1 pound Brussels sprouts, trimmed and quartered
*   (or halved if small)*
1 pound carrots, sliced on a diagonal
2 medium yellow onions, thickly sliced
3 tablespoons avocado oil
1 tablespoon cider vinegar
2 teaspoons garlic powder
Fine sea salt and freshly ground black pepper
4 sprigs fresh rosemary

1. Preheat the oven to 400°F; place two rimmed baking sheets in the oven as it preheats.
2. In a large bowl, combine the Brussels sprouts, carrots, and onions. Drizzle with the oil and vinegar, sprinkle with the garlic powder, and season generously with salt and pepper; toss until all the ingredients are coated.
3. Divide the vegetables between the hot baking sheets, spreading into a single layer, and tuck in the rosemary sprigs in different spots. Roast until the vegetables are tender and caramelized in

spots, 40 to 45 minutes, stirring once or twice during roasting time and switching the baking sheets from top to bottom halfway through. Remove the rosemary sprigs and serve hot, or let cool, cover, and refrigerate to serve cold. (Yield: about 6 cups.)

Per serving: 214 calories, 6 g protein, 27 g carbs, 11 g fat, 9 g fiber

Notes: Be thoughtful when cutting your vegetables; you want them all to cook in the same time frame. Hardier vegetables such as Brussels sprouts or winter squash should be cut smaller than lighter vegetables such as onions.

You can enjoy this as is or drizzle the hot vegetables with your favorite vinaigrette or with Cilantro Pesto *(below) or* Lemon-Herb Tahini Sauce *(page 342).*

If you have leftovers, save them and toss them into a salad, or chop finer and fold into a scramble or frittata.

SAUCES

CILANTRO PESTO

Pesto is traditionally made with basil and pine nuts, but this version gives it an update and a little hint of heat with cilantro, pumpkin seeds, and jalapeño. Leave in the jalapeño seeds if you like it hotter. Hemp seeds help mimic the texture of cheese (this version is dairy-free) and also add a bit of fiber, minerals such as magnesium and zinc, and vitamin E.

Prep: 20 minutes ■ Yield: about 1 cup

2 cups loosely packed fresh cilantro
½ cup loosely packed fresh parsley
⅓ cup roasted, salted pumpkin seeds

¼ cup hemp seeds
1 teaspoon lime zest
¼ cup fresh lime juice
½ medium jalapeño, seeded and diced (about 2 tablespoons)
1 clove garlic, chopped (about 1 teaspoon)
½ cup extra-virgin olive oil
Fine sea salt and freshly ground black pepper

In a food processor, combine the cilantro, parsley, pumpkin seeds, hemp seeds, lime zest and juice, jalapeño, and garlic; pulse several times to chop. With the machine running, drizzle in the oil. Process until the mixture is emulsified and mostly smooth. Taste and season with salt and black pepper. Store leftovers covered in the refrigerator for up to a week.

Per serving (1 tablespoon): 90 calories, 2 g protein, 1 g carbs, 9 g fat, 0 g fiber

Note: You can freeze the pesto. Spoon it into an ice cube tray and freeze, then pop out the cubes and transfer to a freezer bag. Squeeze out the air, seal, and freeze for up to 3 months.

LEMON-HERB TAHINI SAUCE

Tahini—a Middle Eastern sesame seed paste—has enjoyed a renaissance in recent years, showing up in all kinds of recipes both savory and sweet. It's rich and luscious and makes an excellent substitute for peanut butter. Here it's combined with lemon juice and fresh herbs for a flavorful sauce that's full of good nutrition and versatile as well. Make it thick, and it works as a dip. Alternatively, thin it with a little bit of water, reseason, and it becomes a delicious salad dressing or drizzle for steamed or roasted vegetables.

Prep: 25 minutes ■ Cook: 2 minutes ■ Yield: about 1 cup

1 tablespoon olive oil
2 cloves garlic, minced (about 2 teaspoons)
⅓ cup tahini
1 teaspoon lemon zest
¼ cup lemon juice
¼ cup loosely packed fresh parsley
3 tablespoons chopped fresh basil
1 tablespoon chopped fresh mint
½ teaspoon raw honey
Pinch of smoked paprika
⅔ cup hot water
Fine sea salt and freshly ground black pepper

1. In a small unheated skillet, combine the oil and garlic. Turn the heat to low and cook until the mixture begins to sizzle. Allow it to sizzle for 30 seconds undisturbed, then transfer to a small bowl to cool.
2. In a small blender or food processor, combine the tahini, lemon zest and juice, parsley, basil, mint, honey, and paprika; pulse to mix and chop. Add the garlic mixture, pulse a few times, then blend until well combined. Blend in the hot water 1 tablespoon at a time, until the mixture reaches a sauce consistency. Taste and season with salt and pepper.

**Per serving (1 tablespoon): 40 calories, 1 g protein, 2 g carbs,
4 g fat, 1 g fiber**

YOGURT-DILL SAUCE

Greek yogurt and dill are a classic combination, and with good reason—the yogurt's richness and the freshness of dill balance each other beautifully. Have it with vegetables or with lamb, fish, or chicken. It's ready in minutes, so make it for no reason in particular, keep it in the fridge, and you'll see how you can use it to brighten up all kinds of dishes.

Prep: 15 minutes ■ Cook: 2 minutes ■ Yield: about ⅔ cup

2 teaspoons extra-virgin olive oil
2 cloves garlic, minced (about 2 teaspoons)
½ cup plain low-fat Greek yogurt
½ teaspoon lemon zest
1 tablespoon lemon juice
2 tablespoons snipped fresh dill
1 teaspoon chopped fresh mint
Fine sea salt and freshly ground black pepper

1. In a small unheated skillet, combine the oil and garlic. Turn the heat to low and cook until the mixture begins to sizzle. Allow it to sizzle for 30 seconds undisturbed, then transfer to a small bowl to cool.
2. In a medium bowl, whisk together the yogurt, lemon zest and juice, dill, and mint. Fold in the cooled garlic mixture. Taste and season with salt and pepper. Serve, or cover and refrigerate to serve later. (You can make this sauce up to two days ahead; keep covered and refrigerated. Whisk before serving.)

Per serving (1 tablespoon): 19 calories, 1 g protein, 1 g carbs, 1 g fat, 0 g fiber

Note: If you have a personal blender or small food processor and would prefer a smoother sauce, combine all of the ingredients except the salt and pepper, and process until smooth, then taste and season.

SPICY TOMATO SAUCE

Sure, you can buy all manner of jarred tomato sauce—and there's no shame in using a good convenience food. But making your own is surprisingly easy, and you're rewarded with a more complex version that's an instant upgrade. A carrot adds sweetness without sugar (you won't even notice it in the final sauce), and lightly toasting the tomato paste ratchets up the umami. Go light or heavier on the crushed red pepper flakes depending on how much heat you enjoy.

Prep: 15 minutes ■ Cook: 1 hour ■ Yield: about 4 cups

2 tablespoons extra-virgin olive oil
1 small yellow onion, diced (about 1 cup)
Fine sea salt
1 small carrot, shredded (about 1/3 cup)
3 cloves garlic, minced (about 1 tablespoon)
1 tablespoon tomato paste
1/2 to 1 teaspoon crushed red pepper flakes
1 teaspoon dried oregano
3/4 cup chicken or beef bone broth
1 can (28 ounces) crushed tomatoes
Freshly ground black pepper

1. Warm the oil in a large saucepan over medium-low heat. Add the onion, sprinkle with salt, and cook, stirring occasionally, until very tender, 6 to 7 minutes. Add the carrot, sprinkle with salt, and sauté until softened, 1 to 2 minutes. Add the garlic; sauté until fragrant, about 1 minute. Stir in the tomato paste and cook, stirring, until lightly toasted, about 1 minute. Stir in the red pepper flakes and oregano.

2. Add 1/4 cup of the broth; cook, stirring to pull up any browned bits from the bottom of the pan. When nearly all of the broth has evaporated, add the crushed tomatoes and the remaining

½ cup broth. Raise the heat to medium-high and bring just to a boil, then reduce the heat to medium-low, cover, and simmer until the sauce has thickened, 40 to 45 minutes. Taste and season with pepper and additional salt, if needed. Serve, or let cool, cover, and refrigerate.

Per serving (½ cup): 79 calories, 3 g protein, 10 g carbs, 4 g fat, 2 g fiber

Note: If you don't use red pepper flakes, you can swap in harissa (a Middle Eastern chili paste) instead of tomato paste for more heat and a twist on the flavor. Use the same amount, and toast it as you would the tomato paste.

WILD MUSHROOM SAUCE

Mushrooms are such a gift—not only are they flavorful, versatile, and loaded with umami, but they're also good for health, with significant anti-inflammatory, antioxidant power. This classic sauce combines them with shallot, garlic, a touch of white wine, and some bone broth to enhance their flavor. Spoon this sauce on *Herbed Beef Tenderloin* (page 307), *Poached Chicken Breast* (page 312) or *Crisp Roasted Chicken Thighs* (page 314), or use it on any steak, chicken, or fish to make it feel fancy.

Prep: 15 minutes ■ Cook: 15 minutes ■ Yield: about 1 cup

½ to 1 teaspoon arrowroot
1 cup chicken bone broth
1 tablespoon avocado oil
4 ounces wild mushrooms (such as shiitake, oyster, and brown beech), chopped (about 2 cups)
Fine sea salt

1 medium shallot, minced (about ⅓ cup)
2 cloves garlic, minced (about 2 teaspoons)
¼ cup dry white wine
1 tablespoon cold unsalted butter, cut into pieces
1 tablespoon chopped fresh parsley

1. Combine ½ teaspoon arrowroot and ½ teaspoon water in a measuring cup. Whisk in the broth. Warm the oil in a large skillet over medium-high heat. Add the mushrooms, sprinkle with salt, and spread into a single layer. Cook, stirring infrequently and spreading mushrooms out in a single layer, until the mushrooms release their water and begin to turn golden in spots, 4 to 6 minutes. Reduce the heat to medium, add the shallot, sprinkle with salt, and cook, stirring, until tender, 2 to 3 minutes. Add the garlic; sauté until fragrant, about 1 minute.

2. Pour in the wine, and stir to release any browned bits from the bottom of the skillet. Cook, stirring, until the wine has evaporated, about 1 minute. Pour in the broth, bring just to a boil, then reduce the heat and cook, stirring, until the sauce begins to thicken, about 1 minute. Add the butter a piece or two at a time, whisking vigorously, until well incorporated and the sauce has thickened. (If you'd like it thicker, dissolve the remaining ½ teaspoon arrowroot in ½ teaspoon water and whisk it into the sauce. Continue to cook until it thickens.)

3. Remove from the heat. Taste and season with salt. Sprinkle with parsley and serve.

Per serving (2 tablespoons): 51 calories, 2 g protein, 3 g carbs, 3 g fat, 1 g fiber

PURPLE MAGIC SHAKE
(SHAKE + EGGS)

This fun smoothie is a nutrient powerhouse, between the blue spirulina powder, the blackberries, and the pomegranate seeds. Avocado and MCT oil provide healthy fat, and whey lends high-quality protein. But the truly amazing thing about this smoothie is that it tastes just like a Creamsicle—bright orange mixed with creamy vanilla—so unexpected given its intense purple hue. Sip it, or pour it into ice-pop molds and freeze for a post-workout cooldown treat.

Prep: 10 minutes ■ Yield: 1½ cups ■ Serves: 2

¼ *medium ripe avocado*
½ *cup milk of choice (I used almond)*
2 teaspoons blue spirulina powder
1 cup frozen blackberries
¼ *cup pomegranate seeds*
2 teaspoons orange zest
1 tablespoon MCT oil
2 scoops (4 tablespoons) whey protein powder
1 teaspoon vanilla extract
Pinch of fine sea salt
Liquid monkfruit or stevia, optional

Combine the avocado, milk, spirulina powder, blackberries, pomegranate seeds, orange zest, MCT oil, protein powder, vanilla, and salt in a blender; blend until smooth. Taste and sweeten with liquid monkfruit, if needed. Pour into glasses and serve immediately, or pour into ice-pop molds and freeze.

Per serving: 305 calories, 27 g protein, 22 g carbs, 13 g fat, 6 g fiber

NOTES

INTRODUCTION

1. Alyson A. Miller and Sarah J. Spencer, "Obesity and Neuroinflammation: A Pathway to Cognitive Impairment," *Brain, Behavior, and Immunity* 42 (November 2014): 10–21, https://doi.org/10.1016/j.bbi.2014.04.001; Joy Jones Buie, Luke S. Watson, Crystal J. Smith, and Catrina Sims-Robinson, "Obesity-Related Cognitive Impairment: The Role of Endothelial Dysfunction," *Neurobiology of Disease* 132 (December 2019): 104580, https://doi.org/10.1016/j.nbd.2019.104580.

2. Carol Dweck, *Mindset: The New Psychology of Success* (New York: Ballantine, 2016), 16.

CHAPTER 1: SHIFT THE FAT-FOCUSED PARADIGM

1. "Physical Activity Guidelines Resources," ACSM_CMS, accessed May 4, 2023, https://www.acsm.org/education-resources/trending-topics-resources/physical-activity-guidelines.

2. R. R. Wolfe, "Metabolic Interactions between Glucose and Fatty Acids in Humans," *American Journal of Clinical Nutrition* 67, no. 3 (March 1998): 519S–526S, https://doi.org/10.1093/ajcn/67.3.519S.

3. Kim A. Sjøberg, Christian Frøsig, Rasmus Kjøbsted, Lykke Sylow, Maximilian Kleinert, Andrew C. Betik, Christopher S. Shaw, et al., "Exercise Increases Human Skeletal Muscle Insulin Sensitivity via Coordinated Increases in Microvascular Perfusion and Molecular Signaling," *Diabetes* 66, no. 6 (March 2017): 1501–1510, https://doi.org/10.2337/db16-1327.

4. Mohsen Mazidi, Ana M. Valdes, Jose M. Ordovas, Wendy L. Hall, Joan C. Pujol, Jonathan Wolf, George Hadjigeorgiou, et al., "Meal-Induced Inflammation: Postprandial Insights from the Personalised Responses to Dietary Composition Trial (Predict) Study in 1000 Participants," *American Journal of Clinical Nutrition* 114, no. 3 (September 2021): 1028–1038, https://doi.org/10.1093/ajcn/nqab132.

5. Craig S. Stump, Erik J. Henriksen, Yongzhong Wei, and James R. Sowers, "The Metabolic Syndrome: Role of Skeletal Muscle Metabolism," *Annals of Medicine* 38, no. 6 (2006): 389–402, https://doi.org/10.1080/07853890600888413.

6. Ralph A. DeFronzo and Devjit Tripathy, "Skeletal Muscle Insulin Resistance Is the Primary Defect in Type 2 Diabetes," *Diabetes Care* 32, supp. 2 (November 2009): S157–S163, https://doi.org/10.2337/dc09-s302.

7. Hong-Kyu Kim and Chul-Hee Kim, "Quality Matters as Much as Quantity
    of Skeletal Muscle: Clinical Implications of Myosteatosis in Cardiometabolic
    Health," *Endocrinology and Metabolism* 36, no. 6 (December 2021): 1161–1174,
    https://doi.org/10.3803/enm.2021.1348.

8. M. C. K. Severinsen and B. K. Pedersen, "Muscle-Organ Crosstalk: The
    Emerging Roles of Myokines," *Endocrine Reviews* 41, no. 4 (2020): 594–609,
    https://doi.org/10.1210/endrev/bnaa016.

9. Bente Klarlund Pedersen, Thorbjörn C. Åkerström, Anders R. Nielsen, and
    Christian P. Fischer, "Role of Myokines in Exercise and Metabolism," *Journal of
    Applied Physiology* 103, no. 3 (September 2007): 1093–1098, https://doi.org/10
    .1152/japplphysiol.00080.2007.

10. Tsubasa Tomoto, Jie Liu, Benjamin Y. Tseng, Evan P. Pasha, Danilo Cardim,
    Takashi Tarumi, Linda S. Hynan, C. Munro Cullum, and Rong Zhang,
    "One-Year Aerobic Exercise Reduced Carotid Arterial Stiffness and Increased
    Cerebral Blood Flow in Amnestic Mild Cognitive Impairment," *Journal of
    Alzheimer's Disease* 80, no. 2 (March 2021): 841–853, https://doi.org/10.3233/jad
    -201456.

11. P. Z. Liu and R. Nusslock, "Exercise-Mediated Neurogenesis in the
    Hippocampus via BDNF," *Frontiers in Neuroscience* 12 (February 2018), https://
    doi.org/10.3389/fnins.2018.00052.

12. Kirk I. Erickson, Michelle W. Voss, Ruchika Shaurya Prakash, Chandramallika
    Basak, Amanda Szabo, Laura Chaddock, Jennifer S. Kim, et al., "Exercise
    Training Increases Size of Hippocampus and Improves Memory," *Proceedings
    of the National Academy of Sciences* 108, no. 7 (January 31, 2011): 3017–3022,
    https://doi.org/10.1073/pnas.1015950108.

CHAPTER 2: THWART DISEASE

1. Kyle Strimbu and Jorge A. Tavel, "What Are Biomarkers?" *Current Opinion in
    HIV and AIDS* 5, no. 6 (November 2010): 463–466, https://doi.org/10.1097/coh
    .0b013e32833ed177.

2. Pedro L. Valenzuela, Nicola A. Maffiuletti, Gabriella Tringali, Alessandra
    De Col, and Alessandro Sartorio, "Obesity-Associated Poor Muscle Quality:
    Prevalence and Association with Age, Sex, and Body Mass Index," *BMC
    Musculoskeletal Disorders* 21, no. 200 (March 2020), https://doi.org/10.1186
    /s12891-020-03228-y.

3. Eric S. Orwoll, Katherine E. Peters, Marc Hellerstein, Steven R. Cummings,
    William J. Evans, and Peggy M. Cawthon, "The Importance of Muscle versus Fat
    Mass in Sarcopenic Obesity: A Re-evaluation Using D3-Creatine Muscle Mass
    versus DXA Lean Mass Measurements," *Journals of Gerontology: Series A* 75, no. 7
    (July 2020): 1362–1368, https://doi.org/10.1093/gerona/glaa064.

4. "The Innate and Adaptive Immune Systems," NCBI, https://www.ncbi.nlm.nih .gov/books/NBK279396/.

5. Rita Polito, Vincenzo Monda, Ersilia Nigro, Antonietta Messina, Girolamo Di Maio, Maria Teresa Giuliano, Stefania Orrù, et al., "The Important Role of Adiponectin and Orexin-A, Two Key Proteins Improving Healthy Status: Focus on Physical Activity," *Frontiers in Physiology* 11 (April 2020), https://doi.org/10 .3389/fphys.2020.00356.

6. Polito et al., "The Important Role of Adiponectin and Orexin-A."

7. Neil M. Johannsen, Damon L. Swift, William D. Johnson, Vishwa D. Dixit, Conrad P. Earnest, Steven N. Blair, and Timothy S. Church, "Effect of Different Doses of Aerobic Exercise on Total White Blood Cell (WBC) and WBC Subfraction Number in Postmenopausal Women: Results from DREW," *PLOS ONE* 7, no. 2 (February 2012): e31319, https://doi.org/10.1371/journal.pone .0031319.

8. Kassem Sharif, Abdulla Watad, Nicola Luigi Bragazzi, Micheal Lichtbroun, Howard Amital, and Yehuda Shoenfeld, "Physical Activity and Autoimmune Diseases: Get Moving and Manage the Disease," *Autoimmunity Reviews* 17, no. 1 (January 2018): 53–72, https://doi.org/10.1016/j.autrev.2017.11.010.

9. Luiz Augusto Perandini, Ana Lúcia de Sá-Pinto, Hamilton Roschel, Fabiana Braga Benatti, Fernanda Rodrigues Lima, Eloisa Bonfá, and Bruno Gualano, "Exercise as a Therapeutic Tool to Counteract Inflammation and Clinical Symptoms in Autoimmune Rheumatic Diseases," *Autoimmunity Reviews* 12, no. 2 (December 2012): 218–224, https://doi.org/10.1016/j.autrev.2012.06.007.

10. "Global Cancer Facts & Figures," American Cancer Society, https://www.cancer .org/research/cancer-facts-statistics/global.html.

11. "Diet and Cancer Prevention," *Tufts Health & Nutrition Letter*, December 1, 2020, https://www.nutritionletter.tufts.edu/special-reports/diet-and-cancer -prevention/.

12. Veronica Wendy Setiawan, Hannah P. Yang, Malcolm C. Pike, Susan E. McCann, Herbert Yu, Yong-Bing Xiang, Alicja Wolk, et al., "Type I and II Endometrial Cancers: Have They Different Risk Factors?" *Journal of Clinical Oncology* 31, no. 20 (June 2013): 2607–2618, https:// doi.org/10.1200/jco.2012.48.2596.

13. Cathrine Hoyo, Michael B. Cook, Farin Kamangar, Neal D. Freedman, David C. Whiteman, Leslie Bernstein, Linda M. Brown, et al., "Body Mass Index in Relation to Oesophageal and Oesophagogastric Junction Adenocarcinomas: A Pooled Analysis from the International Beacon Consortium," *International Journal of Epidemiology* 41, no. 6 (November 2012): 1706–1718, https://doi.org /10.1093/ije/dys176.

14. Yi Chen, Lingxiao Liu, Xiaolin Wang, Jianhua Wang, Zhiping Yan, Jieming Cheng, Gaoquan Gong, and Guoping Li, "Body Mass Index and Risk of Gastric

Cancer: A Meta-Analysis of a Population with More Than Ten Million from 24 Prospective Studies," *Cancer Epidemiology, Biomarkers & Prevention* 22, no. 8 (May 2013): 1395–1408, https://doi.org/10.1158/1055-9965.epi-13-0042.

15. Jeanine M. Genkinger, Donna Spiegelman, Kristin E. Anderson, Leslie Bernstein, Piet A. van den Brandt, Eugenia E. Calle, Dallas R. English, et al., "A Pooled Analysis of 14 Cohort Studies of Anthropometric Factors and Pancreatic Cancer Risk," *International Journal of Cancer* 129, no. 7 (March 2011): 1708–1717, https://doi.org/10.1002/ijc.25794.

16. Yanlei Ma, Yongzhi Yang, Feng Wang, Peng Zhang, Chenzhang Shi, Yang Zou, and Huanlong Qin, "Obesity and Risk of Colorectal Cancer: A Systematic Review of Prospective Studies," *PLOS ONE* 8, no. 1 (January 2013), https://doi.org/10.1371/journal.pone.0053916.

17. "Diet, Nutrition, Physical Activity and Gallbladder Cancer," World Cancer Research Fund, https://www.wcrf.org/wp-content/uploads/2021/02/gall bladder-cancer-report.pdf; Liqing Li, Yong Gan, Wenzheng Li, Chunmei Wu, and Zuxun Lu, "Overweight, Obesity and the Risk of Gallbladder and Extrahepatic Bile Duct Cancers: A Meta-Analysis of Observational Studies," *Obesity* 24, no. 8 (July 2016): 1786–1802, https://doi.org/10.1002/oby.21505.

18. Andrew G. Renehan, Margaret Tyson, Matthias Egger, Richard F. Heller, and Marcel Zwahlen, "Body-Mass Index and Incidence of Cancer: A Systematic Review and Meta-Analysis of Prospective Observational Studies," *The Lancet* 371, no. 9612 (February 2008): 569–578, https://doi.org/10.1016/s0140-6736(08)60269-x.

19. Mark F. Munsell, Brian L. Sprague, Donald A. Berry, Gary Chisholm, and Amy Trentham-Dietz, "Body Mass Index and Breast Cancer Risk According to Postmenopausal Estrogen-Progestin Use and Hormone Receptor Status," *Epidemiologic Reviews* 36, no. 1 (2014): 114–136, https://doi.org/10.1093/epirev/mxt010.

20. "Ovarian Cancer and Body Size: Individual Participant Meta-Analysis Including 25,157 Women with Ovarian Cancer from 47 Epidemiological Studies," *PLOS Medicine* 9, no. 4 (April 2012), https://doi.org/10.1371/journal.pmed.1001200.

21. Lee W. Jones, Laurel A. Habel, Erin Weltzien, Adrienne Castillo, Dipti Gupta, Candyce H. Kroenke, Marilyn L. Kwan, et al., "Exercise and Risk of Cardiovascular Events in Women with Nonmetastatic Breast Cancer," *Journal of Clinical Oncology* 34, no. 23 (August 2016): 2743–2749, https://doi.org/10.1200/jco.2015.65.6603.

22. Michael J. Tisdale, "The 'Cancer Cachectic Factor,'" *Supportive Care in Cancer* 11, no. 2 (February 2003): 73–78, https://doi.org/10.1007/s00520-002-0408-6.

23. Josep M. Argilés, Sílvia Busquets, Britta Stemmler, and Francisco J. López-Soriano, "Cancer Cachexia: Understanding the Molecular Basis," *Nature Reviews Cancer* 14, no. 11 (October 2014): 754–762, https://doi.org/10.1038/nrc3829.

24. Eric J. Roeland, Kari Bohlke, Vickie E. Baracos, Eduardo Bruera, Egidio del Fabbro, Suzanne Dixon, Marie Fallon, et al., "Management of Cancer Cachexia: ASCO Guideline," *Journal of Clinical Oncology* 38, no. 21 (July 2020): 2438–2453, https://doi.org/10.1200/jco.20.00611.

25. R. Donato et al., "Functions of S100 Proteins," *Current Molecular Medicine* 13, no. 1 (January 2013): 24–57, https://pubmed.ncbi.nlm.nih.gov/22834835/.

26. Justin P. Hardee, Melissa J. Puppa, Dennis K. Fix, Song Gao, Kimbell L. Hetzler, Ted A. Bateman, and James A. Carson, "The Effect of Radiation Dose on Mouse Skeletal Muscle Remodeling," *Radiology and Oncology* 48, no. 3 (July 2014): 247–256, https://doi.org/10.2478/raon-2014-0025.

27. Georgios Mavropalias, Marc Sim, Dennis R. Taaffe, Daniel A. Galvão, Nigel Spry, William J. Kraemer, Keijo Häkkinen, and Robert U. Newton, "Exercise Medicine for Cancer Cachexia: Targeted Exercise to Counteract Mechanisms and Treatment Side Effects," *Journal of Cancer Research and Clinical Oncology* 148, no. 6 (January 2022): 1389–1406, https://doi.org/10.1007/s00432-022-03927-0.

28. Mitsuharu Matsumoto, Yusuke Kitada, and Yuji Naito, "Endothelial Function Is Improved by Inducing Microbial Polyamine Production in the Gut: A Randomized Placebo-Controlled Trial," *Nutrients* 11, no. 5 (May 2019): 1188, https://doi.org/10.3390/nu11051188.

29. Kristin L. Campbell, Kerri M. Winters-Stone, Joachim Wiskemann, Anne M. May, Anna L. Schwartz, Kerry S. Courneya, David S. Zucker, et al., "Exercise Guidelines for Cancer Survivors: Consensus Statement from International Multidisciplinary Roundtable," *Medicine & Science in Sports & Exercise* 51, no. 11 (November 2019): 2375–2390, https://doi.org/10.1249/mss.0000000000002116.

30. Fatma Alzahraa H. Kamel, Maged A. Basha, Ashwag S. Alsharidah, and Amr B. Salama, "Resistance Training Impact on Mobility, Muscle Strength and Lean Mass in Pancreatic Cancer Cachexia: A Randomized Controlled Trial," *Clinical Rehabilitation* 34, no. 11 (July 2020): 1391–1399, https://doi.org/10.1177/0269215520941912.

31. Mavropalias et al., "Exercise Medicine for Cancer Cachexia."

32. Mavropalias et al., "Exercise Medicine for Cancer Cachexia."

33. Manit Saeteaw, Phitjira Sanguanboonyaphong, Jukapun Yoodee, Kaitlyn Craft, Ratree Sawangjit, Nuttapong Ngamphaiboon, Prapimporn Chattranukulchai Shantavasinkul, Suphat Subongkot, and Nathorn Chaiyakunapruk, "Efficacy and Safety of Pharmacological Cachexia Interventions: Systematic Review and Network Meta-Analysis," *BMJ Supportive & Palliative Care* 11, no. 1 (November 2020): 75–85, https://doi.org/10.1136/bmjspcare-2020-002601.

34. Kathryn H. Schmitz, Anna M. Campbell, Martijn M. Stuiver, Bernardine M. Pinto, Anna L. Schwartz, G. Stephen Morris, Jennifer A. Ligibel, et al., "Exercise Is Medicine in Oncology: Engaging Clinicians to Help Patients Move through

Cancer," *CA: A Cancer Journal for Clinicians* 69, no. 6 (October 2019): 468–484, https://doi.org/10.3322/caac.21579.

35. Martin Prince, Renata Bryce, Emiliano Albanese, Anders Wimo, Wagner Ribeiro, and Cleusa P. Ferri, "The Global Prevalence of Dementia: A Systematic Review and Metaanalysis," *Alzheimer's & Dementia* 9, no. 1 (January 2013): 63, https://doi.org/10.1016/j.jalz.2012.11.007.

36. Subbiah Pugazhenthi, Limei Qin, and P. Hemachandra Reddy, "Common Neurodegenerative Pathways in Obesity, Diabetes, and Alzheimer's Disease," *Biochimica et Biophysica Acta (BBA)—Molecular Basis of Disease* 1863, no. 5 (May 2017): 1037–1045, https://doi.org/10.1016/j.bbadis.2016.04.017.

37. T. Kelly, W. Yang, C.-S. Chen, K. Reynolds, and J. He, "Global Burden of Obesity in 2005 and Projections to 2030," *International Journal of Obesity* 32, no. 9 (July 2008): 1431–1437, https://doi.org/10.1038/ijo.2008.102.

38. Mika Kivimäki, Ritva Luukkonen, G. David Batty, Jane E. Ferrie, Jaana Pentti, Solja T. Nyberg, Martin J. Shipley, et al., "Body Mass Index and Risk of Dementia: Analysis of Individual-Level Data from 1.3 Million Individuals," *Alzheimer's & Dementia* 14, no. 5 (November 2017): 601–609, https://doi.org/10.1016/j.jalz.2017.09.016.

39. "Evidence Profile: Weight Reduction and Cognitive Decline or Dementia," Risk Reduction of Cognitive Decline and Dementia: WHO Guidelines, https://www.ncbi.nlm.nih.gov/books/NBK542803/.

40. Emily Balcetis, *Clearer, Closer, Better: How Successful People See the World* (New York: Ballantine, 2020).

CHAPTER 3: BULLETPROOF YOUR CHANGING BODY FOR STRENGTH AT EVERY AGE

1. "New Research Uncovers Concerning Increases in Youth Living with Diabetes in the U.S.," Centers for Disease Control and Prevention, August 24, 2021, https://www.cdc.gov/media/releases/2021/p0824-youth-diabetes.html.

2. Laura Reiley, "USDA Announces Rigorous New School Nutrition Standards," *Washington Post*, February 3, 2023, https://www.washingtonpost.com/business/2023/02/03/school-meals-dietary-guidelines/.

3. Mark D. Peterson, Peng Zhang, William A. Saltarelli, Paul S. Visich, and Paul M. Gordon, "Low Muscle Strength Thresholds for the Detection of Cardiometabolic Risk in Adolescents," *American Journal of Preventive Medicine* 50, no. 5 (May 2016): 593–599, https://doi.org/10.1016/j.amepre.2015.09.019.

4. Laura D. Brown, "Endocrine Regulation of Fetal Skeletal Muscle Growth: Impact on Future Metabolic Health," *Journal of Endocrinology* 221, no. 2 (February 2014): 13–29, https://doi.org/10.1530/joe-13-0567.

5. Marcus Moberg, Malene E. Lindholm, Stefan M. Reitzner, Björn Ekblom, Carl-Johan Sundberg, and Niklas Psilander, "Exercise Induces Different Molecular Responses in Trained and Untrained Human Muscle," *Medicine & Science in Sports & Exercise* 52, no. 8 (August 2020): 1679–1690, https://doi.org/10.1249/mss.0000000000002310.

6. Paul R. Stricker, Avery D. Faigenbaum, Teri M. McCambridge, Cynthia R. LaBella, M. Alison Brooks, Greg Canty, Alex B. Diamond, et al., "Resistance Training for Children and Adolescents," *Pediatrics* 145, no. 6 (June 2020), https://doi.org/10.1542/peds.2020-1011.

7. Joshua L. Hudson, Jamie I. Baum, Eva C. Diaz, and Elisabet Børsheim, "Dietary Protein Requirements in Children: Methods for Consideration," *Nutrients* 13, no. 5 (May 2021): 1554, https://doi.org/10.3390/nu13051554.

8. Minghua Tang, "Protein Intake during the First Two Years of Life and Its Association with Growth and Risk of Overweight," *International Journal of Environmental Research and Public Health* 15, no. 8 (August 2018): 1742, https://doi.org/10.3390/ijerph15081742.

9. Masoud Rahmati, John J. McCarthy, and Fatemeh Malakoutinia, "Myonuclear Permanence in Skeletal Muscle Memory: A Systematic Review and Meta-Analysis of Human and Animal Studies," *Journal of Cachexia, Sarcopenia and Muscle* 13, no. 5 (August 2022): 2276–2297, https://doi.org/10.1002/jcsm.13043.

10. Kristian Gundersen, "Muscle Memory and a New Cellular Model for Muscle Atrophy and Hypertrophy," *Journal of Experimental Biology* 219, no. 2 (January 2016): 235–242, https://doi.org/10.1242/jeb.124495.

11. A. A. Sayer, H. Syddall, H. Martin, H. Patel, D. Baylis, and C. Cooper, "The Developmental Origins of Sarcopenia," *Journal of Nutrition Health and Aging* 12, no. 7 (August 2008): 427–432, https://doi.org/10.1007/bf02982703.

12. Barbara E. Kahn and Robert E. Brannigan, "Obesity and Male Infertility," *Current Opinion in Urology* 27, no. 5 (September 2017): 441–445, https://doi.org/10.1097/mou.0000000000000417.

13. Thibault Sutter, Hechmi Toumi, Antoine Valery, Rawad El Hage, Antonio Pinti, and Eric Lespessailles, "Relationships between Muscle Mass, Strength and Regional Bone Mineral Density in Young Men," *PLOS ONE* 14, no. 3 (March 2019), https://doi.org/10.1371/journal.pone.0213681.

14. W. Ombelet, I. Cooke, S. Dyer, G. Serour, and P. Devroey, "Infertility and the Provision of Infertility Medical Services in Developing Countries," *Human Reproduction Update* 14, no. 6 (September 2008): 605–621, https://doi.org/10.1093/humupd/dmn042.

15. A. B. Jose-Miller, J. W. Boyden, and K. A. Frey, "Infertility," *American Family Physician* 75 (March 2007): 849–856.

16. E. Silvestris, G. de Pergola, R. Rosania, and G. Loverro, "Obesity as Disruptor of the Female Fertility," *Reproductive Biology and Endocrinology* 16, no. 22 (March

2018), https://doi.org/10.1186/s12958-018-0336-z.; L. Currie, "Fall and Injury Prevention," in *Patient Safety and Quality: An Evidence-Based Handbook for Nurses*, ed. R. G. Hughes (Rockville, MD: Agency for Healthcare Research and Quality, 2008), chap. 10, https://pubmed.ncbi.nlm.nih.gov/21328752/.

17. Laura E. McBreairty, Philip D. Chilibeck, Julianne J. Gordon, Donna R. Chizen, and Gordon A. Zello, "Polycystic Ovary Syndrome Is a Risk Factor for Sarcopenic Obesity: A Case Control Study," *BMC Endocrine Disorders* 19, no. 70 (July 2019), https://doi.org/10.1186/s12902-019-0381-4.

18. Tara McDonnell, Leanne Cussen, Marie McIlroy, and Michael W. O'Reilly, "Characterizing Skeletal Muscle Dysfunction in Women with Polycystic Ovary Syndrome," *Therapeutic Advances in Endocrinology and Metabolism* 13 (January 2022), https://doi.org/10.1177/20420188221113140.

19. Solvejg L. Hansen, Pernille F. Svendsen, Jacob F. Jeppesen, Louise D. Hoeg, Nicoline R. Andersen, Jonas M. Kristensen, Lisbeth Nilas, et al., "Molecular Mechanisms in Skeletal Muscle Underlying Insulin Resistance in Women Who Are Lean with Polycystic Ovary Syndrome," *Journal of Clinical Endocrinology & Metabolism* 104, no. 5 (December 2018): 1841–1854, https://doi.org/10.1210/jc .2018-01771.

20. Ulla Kampmann, Sine Knorr, Jens Fuglsang, and Per Ovesen, "Determinants of Maternal Insulin Resistance during Pregnancy: An Updated Overview," *Journal of Diabetes Research* 2019 (November 2019): 1–9, https://doi.org/10.1155/2019 /5320156.

21. "Gestational Diabetes," American Diabetes Association, https://diabetes.org /diabetes/gestational-diabetes.

22. H. David McIntyre, Patrick Catalano, Cuilin Zhang, Gernot Desoye, Elisabeth R. Mathiesen, and Peter Damm, "Gestational Diabetes Mellitus," *Nature Reviews Disease Primers* 5, no. 1 (July 2019), https://doi.org/10.1038/s41572-019-0098-8.

23. Raul Narvaez-Sanchez, Juan C. Calderón, Gloria Vega, Maria Camila Trillos, and Sara Ospina, "Skeletal Muscle as a Protagonist in the Pregnancy Metabolic Syndrome," *Medical Hypotheses* 126 (May 2019): 26–37, https://doi.org/10.1016 /j.mehy.2019.02.049.

24. Narvaez-Sanchez et al., "Skeletal Muscle."

25. Yaping Xie, Huifen Zhao, Meijing Zhao, Huibin Huang, Chunhong Liu, Fengfeng Huang, and Jingjing Wu, "Effects of Resistance Exercise on Blood Glucose Level and Pregnancy Outcome in Patients with Gestational Diabetes Mellitus: A Randomized Controlled Trial," *BMJ Open Diabetes Research & Care* 10, no. 2 (April 2022), https://doi.org/10.1136/bmjdrc-2021-002622.

26. Behzad Hajizadeh Maleki, Bakhtyar Tartibian, and Mohammad Chehrazi, "Effectiveness of Exercise Training on Male Factor Infertility: A Systematic Review and Network Meta-Analysis," *Sports Health: A*

Multidisciplinary Approach 14, no. 4 (November 2021): 508–517, https://doi.org/10.1177/19417381211055399.

27. Behzad Hajizadeh Maleki and Bakhtyar Tartibian, "Resistance Exercise Modulates Male Factor Infertility through Anti-Inflammatory and Antioxidative Mechanisms in Infertile Men: A RCT," *Life Sciences* 203 (June 2018): 150–160, https://doi.org/10.1016/j.lfs.2018.04.039.

28. Nicholas A. Christakis and James H. Fowler, "The Spread of Obesity in a Large Social Network over 32 Years," *New England Journal of Medicine* 357, no. 4 (July 2007): 370–79, https://doi.org/10.1056/nejmsa066082.

29. Kirk L. English and Douglas Paddon-Jones, "Protecting Muscle Mass and Function in Older Adults during Bed Rest," *Current Opinion in Clinical Nutrition and Metabolic Care* 13, no. 1 (January 2010): 34–39, https://doi.org/10.1097/mco.0b013e328333aa66; Mauro Zamboni et al., "Sarcopenic Obesity: A New Category of Obesity in the Elderly," *Nutrition, Metabolism and Cardiovascular Diseases* 18, no. 5 (2008): 388–395.

30. Micah J. Drummond, Jared M. Dickinson, Christopher S. Fry, Dillon K. Walker, David M. Gundermann, Paul T. Reidy, Kyle L. Timmerman, et al., "Bed Rest Impairs Skeletal Muscle Amino Acid Transporter Expression, mtorc1 Signaling, and Protein Synthesis in Response to Essential Amino Acids in Older Adults," *American Journal of Physiology-Endocrinology and Metabolism* 302, no. 9 (May 2012), https://doi.org/10.1152/ajpendo.00603.2011.

31. David M. Almeida, Jonathan Rush, Jacqueline Mogle, Jennifer R. Piazza, Eric Cerino, and Susan T. Charles, "Longitudinal Change in Daily Stress across 20 Years of Adulthood: Results from the National Study of Daily Experiences," *Developmental Psychology* 59, no. 3 (March 2023): 515–523, https://doi.org/10.1037/dev0001469; C. Allen, P. Glasziou, and C. Del Mar, "Bed Rest: A Potentially Harmful Treatment Needing More Careful Evaluation," *The Lancet* 354, no. 9186 (October 1999): 1229–1233, https://doi.org/10.1016/s0140-6736(98)10063-6.

32. Sumito Ogawa, Mitsutaka Yakabe, and Masahiro Akishita, "Age-Related Sarcopenia and Its Pathophysiological Bases," *Inflammation and Regeneration* 36, no. 1 (September 2016), https://doi.org/10.1186/s41232-016-0022-5.

33. Nkechinyere Chidi-Ogbolu and Keith Baar, "Effect of Estrogen on Musculoskeletal Performance and Injury Risk," *Frontiers in Physiology* 9 (January 2019), https://doi.org/10.3389/fphys.2018.01834.

34. William Chen, David Datzkiw, and Michael A. Rudnicki, "Satellite Cells in Ageing: Use It or Lose It," *Open Biology* 10, no. 5 (May 2020), https://doi.org/10.1098/rsob.200048; Mitsutaka Yakabe, Sumito Ogawa, and Masahiro Akishita, "Clinical Manifestations and Pathophysiology of Sarcopenia," *Biomedical Sciences* 1, no. 2 (July 2015): 10–17.

35. Chidi-Ogbolu and Baar, "Effect of Estrogen."

36. Chen at el., "Satellite Cells."

37. Currie, "Fall and Injury."

38. Pedro Lopez, Ronei Silveira Pinto, Regis Radaelli, Anderson Rech, Rafael
Grazioli, Mikel Izquierdo, and Eduardo Lusa Cadore, "Benefits of Resistance
Training in Physically Frail Elderly: A Systematic Review," *Aging Clinical and
Experimental Research* 30, no. 8 (November 2017): 889–899, https://doi.org/10
.1007/s40520-017-0863-z.

39. M. Sun, L. Min, N. Xu, L. Huang, and X. Li, "The Effect of Exercise
Intervention on Reducing the Fall Risk in Older Adults: A Meta-Analysis
of Randomized Controlled Trials," *International Journal of Environmental
Research and Public Health*, 18, no.23 (2021): 12562, https://doi.org/10.3390/
ijerph182312562.

CHAPTER 4: SLAM-DUNK SUCCESS WITH NUTRITIONAL SCIENCE

1. Dariush Mozaffarian, Irwin Rosenberg, and Ricardo Uauy, "History of Modern
Nutrition Science—Implications for Current Research, Dietary Guidelines, and
Food Policy," *BMJ* (June 2018), https://doi.org/10.1136/bmj.k2392.

2. Arne Astrup, Faidon Magkos, Dennis M. Bier, J. Thomas Brenna, Marcia C. de
Oliveira Otto, James O. Hill, Janet C. King, et al., "Saturated Fats and Health:
A Reassessment and Proposal for Food-Based Recommendations," *Journal of the
American College of Cardiology* 76, no. 7 (August 2020): 844–857, https://doi.org
/10.1016/j.jacc.2020.05.077.

3. Jeffrey Heydu, "Cultural Modeling in Two Eras of U.S. Food Protest:
Grahamites (1830s) and Organic Advocates (1960s–70s)," *Social Problems* 58,
no. 3 (August 2011): 461–487, https://www.academia.edu/21735004/Cultural
_Modeling_in_Two_Eras_of_U_S_Food_Protest_Grahamites_1830s_and
_Organic_Advocates_1960s_70s_.

4. "World War II Veterans by the Numbers," VA Fact Sheet, https://dig.abclocal.go
.com/ktrk/ktrk_120710_WWIIvetsfactsheet.pdf.

5. Cari Romm, "The World War II Campaign to Bring Organ Meats to the Dinner
Table," *The Atlantic*, September 25, 2014, https://www.theatlantic.com/health
/archive/2014/09/the-world-war-ii-campaign-to-bring-organ-meats-to-the-dinner
-table/380737/.

6. Catherine Price, "The Age of Scurvy," *Distillations*, August 14, 2017, https://www
.sciencehistory.org/distillations/the-age-of-scurvy.

7. "Divorce Rate in Maine Correlates with per Capita Consumption of Margarine
(US)," Spurious Correlations, https://www.tylervigen.com/view_correlation?id=
1703.

8. Julia Faria, "PepsiCo: Ad Spend in the U.S. 2014–2021," Statista, January 6,
2023, https://www.statista.com/statistics/585833/pepsico-ad-spend-usa/#:~:text=

In%202021%2C%20PepsiCo%20invested%201.96,increased%20by%20around
%2012%20percent.

9. Ronald W. Ward, "Commodity Checkoff Programs and Generic Advertising," *Choices* 21, no. 2 (2006): 55–60, https://www.choicesmagazine.org/2006 -2/checkoff/2006-2-02.htm.

10. "Research & Promotion Programs," USDA, https://www.ams.usda.gov/rules -regulations/research-promotion.

11. Justin McCarthy and Scott DeKoster, "Nearly One in Four in U.S. Have Cut Back on Eating Meat," Gallup, January 27, 2020, https://news.gallup.com/poll /282779/nearly-one-four-cut-back-eating-meat.aspx.

12. "Livestock and Meat Domestic Data," USDA, https://www.ers.usda.gov/data -products/livestock-and-meat-domestic-data/.

13. Florent Vieux, Didier Rémond, Jean-Louis Peyraud, and Nicole Darmon, "Approximately Half of Total Protein Intake by Adults Must Be Animal-Based to Meet Nonprotein, Nutrient-Based Recommendations, with Variations Due to Age and Sex," *Journal of Nutrition* 152, no. 11 (November 2022): 2514–2525, https://doi.org/10.1093/jn/nxac150.

14. Joséphine Gehring, Mathilde Touvier, Julia Baudry, Chantal Julia, Camille Buscail, Bernard Srour, Serge Hercberg, Sandrine Péneau, Emmanuelle Kesse-Guyot, and Benjamin Allès, "Consumption of Ultra-Processed Foods by Pesco-Vegetarians, Vegetarians, and Vegans: Associations with Duration and Age at Diet Initiation," *Journal of Nutrition* 151, no. 1 (January 2021): 120–131, https:// doi.org/10.1093/jn/nxaa196.

15. "Food Availability and Consumption," USDA, https://www.ers.usda.gov/data -products/ag-and-food-statistics-charting-the-essentials/food-availability-and -consumption/.

16. Heather J. Leidy, Peter M. Clifton, Arne Astrup, Thomas P. Wycherley, Margriet S. Westerterp-Plantenga, Natalie D. Luscombe-Marsh, Stephen C. Woods, and Richard D. Mattes, "The Role of Protein in Weight Loss and Maintenance," *American Journal of Clinical Nutrition* 101, no. 6 (June 2015): 1320S–1329S, https://doi.org/10.3945/ajcn.114.084038.

17. Zhilei Shan, Colin D. Rehm, Gail Rogers, Mengyuan Ruan, Dong D. Wang, Frank B. Hu, Dariush Mozaffarian, Fang Fang Zhang, and Shilpa N. Bhupathiraju, "Trends in Dietary Carbohydrate, Protein, and Fat Intake and Diet Quality among US Adults, 1999–2016," *JAMA* 322, no. 12 (September 2019): 1178, https://doi.org/10.1001/jama.2019.13771.

18. Stephan van Vliet, James R. Bain, Michael J. Muehlbauer, Frederick D. Provenza, Scott L. Kronberg, Carl F. Pieper, and Kim M. Huffman, "A Metabolomics Comparison of Plant-Based Meat and Grass-Fed Meat Indicates Large Nutritional Differences Despite Comparable Nutrition Facts Panels," *Scientific Reports* 11, no. 13828 (July 2021), https://doi.org/10.1038/s41598-021-93100-3.

19. Frédéric Leroy, Fabien Abraini, Ty Beal, Paula Dominguez-Salas, Pablo Gregorini, Pablo Manzano, Jason Rowntree, and Stephan van Vliet, "Animal Board Invited Review: Animal Source Foods in Healthy, Sustainable, and Ethical Diets—An Argument against Drastic Limitation of Livestock in the Food System," *Animal* 16, no. 3 (March 2022): 100457, https://doi.org/10.1016/j.animal.2022.100457.

20. C. Biltekoff, *Eating Right in America: The Cultural Politics of Food and Health* (Durham, NC: Duke University Press, 2013); Frédéric Leroy and Adele H. Hite, "The Place of Meat in Dietary Policy: An Exploration of the Animal/Plant Divide," *Meat and Muscle Biology* 4, no. 2 (July 2020), https://doi.org/10.22175/mmb.9456.

21. Frédéric Leroy, "Meat as a Pharmakon: An Exploration of the Biosocial Complexities of Meat Consumption," in *Advances in Food and Nutrition Research*, vol. 87, ed. Fidel Toldrá (Cambridge, MA: Academic Press, 2019), 409–446.

22. Maria Chiorando, "Plant Based Brand Oatly Addresses Controversy over Selling Oat Residue to Pig Farm," *Plant Based News*, October 1, 2020, https://plantbasednews.org/lifestyle/plant-based-oatly-addresses-controversy-selling-oat-residue-pig-farm/.

23. Frank Mitloehner, "Livestock's Contributions to Climate Change: Facts and Fiction," University of California, https://cekern.ucanr.edu/files/256942.pdf.

24. Robin R. White and Mary Beth Hall, "Nutritional and Greenhouse Gas Impacts of Removing Animals from US Agriculture," *Proceedings of the National Academy of Sciences* 114, no. 48 (November 2017): E10301–E10308, https://doi.org/10.1073/pnas.1707322114.

25. "Inventory of U.S. Greenhouse Gas Emissions and Sinks," Environmental Protection Agency, https://www.epa.gov/ghgemissions/inventory-us-greenhouse-gas-emissions-and-sinks.

26. White and Hall, "Nutritional and Greenhouse Gas Impacts."

27. White and Hall, "Nutritional and Greenhouse Gas Impacts."

28. W. R. Teague, "Forages and Pastures Symposium: Cover Crops in Livestock Production: Whole-System Approach: Managing Grazing to Restore Soil Health and Farm Livelihoods," *Journal of Animal Science* 96, no. 4 (February 2018): 1519–1530, https://doi.org/10.1093/jas/skx060.

29. R. Lal, "Soil Erosion Impact on Agronomic Productivity and Environment Quality," *Critical Reviews in Plant Sciences* 17, no. 4 (July 1998): 319–464, https://doi.org/10.1080/07352689891304249.

30. "Sources of Greenhouse Gas Emissions," Environmental Protection Agency, https://www.epa.gov/ghgemissions/sources-greenhouse-gas-emissions.

31. Lal, "Soil Erosion Impact."

32. "Adult Obesity Facts," Centers for Disease Control and Prevention, https://www .cdc.gov/obesity/data/adult.html.

33. Viktor E. Frankl, Ilse Lasch, Harold S. Kushner, and William J. Winslade, *Man's Search for Meaning* (Boston: Beacon, 2019).

CHAPTER 5: PROTEIN: MORE THAN JUST A MACRONUTRIENT

1. Donald K. Layman, "Dietary Guidelines Should Reflect New Understandings about Adult Protein Needs," *Nutrition & Metabolism* 6, no. 1 (March 2009): 12, https://doi.org/10.1186/1743-7075-6-12.

2. M. C. Devries, A. Sithamparapillai, K. S. Brimble, L. Banfield, R. W. Morton, and S. M. Phillips, "Changes in Kidney Function Do Not Differ between Healthy Adults Consuming Higher- Compared with Lower- or Normal-Protein Diets: A Systematic Review and Meta-Analysis," *Journal of Nutrition* 148, no. 11 (2018): 1760–1775, https://doi.org/10.1093/jn/nxy197.

3. M. E. Van Elswyk, C. A. Weatherford, and S. H. McNeill, "A Systematic Review of Renal Health in Healthy Individuals Associated with Protein Intake above the US Recommended Daily Allowance in Randomized Controlled Trials and Observational Studies," *Advances in Nutrition* 9, no. 4 (2018): 404–418, https:// doi.org/10.1093/advances/nmy026.

4. Jess A. Gwin, David D. Church, Robert R. Wolfe, Arny A. Ferrando, and Stefan M. Pasiakos, "Muscle Protein Synthesis and Whole-Body Protein Turnover Responses to Ingesting Essential Amino Acids, Intact Protein, and Protein-Containing Mixed Meals with Considerations for Energy Deficit," *Nutrients* 12, no. 8 (August 2020): 2457, https://doi.org/10.3390/nu12082457.

5. Louise A. Berner, Gabriel Becker, Maxwell Wise, and Jimmy Doi, "Characterization of Dietary Protein among Older Adults in the United States: Amount, Animal Sources, and Meal Patterns," *Journal of the Academy of Nutrition and Dietetics* 113, no. 6 (June 2013): 809–815, https://doi.org/10.1016/j.jand.2013 .01.014.

6. Ulrika J. Gunnerud, Cornelia Heinzle, Jens J. Holst, Elin M. Östman, and Inger M. Björck, "Effects of Pre-Meal Drinks with Protein and Amino Acids on Glycemic and Metabolic Responses at a Subsequent Composite Meal," *PLOS ONE* 7, no. 9 (September 2012), https://doi.org/10.1371/journal.pone.0044731.

7. Ralf Jäger, Chad M. Kerksick, Bill I. Campbell, Paul J. Cribb, Shawn D. Wells, Tim M. Skwiat, Martin Purpura, et al., "International Society of Sports Nutrition Position Stand: Protein and Exercise," *Journal of the International Society of Sports Nutrition* 14, no. 1 (January 2017), https://doi.org/10.1186 /s12970-017-0177-8.

8. Mathijs Drummen, Lea Tischmann, Blandine Gatta-Cherifi, Tanja Adam, and Margriet Westerterp-Plantenga, "Dietary Protein and Energy Balance in Relation

to Obesity and Co-Morbidities," *Frontiers in Endocrinology* 9 (August 2018), https://doi.org/10.3389/fendo.2018.00443.

9. Dr. Heather Leidy has done some pivotal work in this area. Heather J. Leidy, Richard D. Mattes, and Wayne W. Campbell, "Effects of Acute and Chronic Protein Intake on Metabolism, Appetite, and Ghrelin during Weight Loss," *Obesity* 15, no. 5 (2007): 1215–1225, https://doi.org/10.1038/oby.2007.143.

CHAPTER 6: CARBOHYDRATES AND DIETARY FATS: DEMYSTIFYING THE DARLINGS OF NUTRITIONAL SCIENCE

1. David S. Ludwig and Cara B. Ebbeling, "The Carbohydrate-Insulin Model of Obesity," *JAMA Internal Medicine* 178, no. 8 (August 2018): 1098, https://doi.org/10.1001/jamainternmed.2018.2933.

2. Shan et al., "Trends in Dietary Carbohydrate, Protein, and Fat Intake."

3. Mary C. Gannon and Frank Q. Nuttall, "Amino Acid Ingestion and Glucose Metabolism—A Review," *IUBMB Life* 62, no. 9 (September 2010): 660–668, https://doi.org/10.1002/iub.375.

4. S. Sonia, F. Witjaksono, and R. Ridwan, "Effect of Cooling of Cooked White Rice on Resistant Starch Content and Glycemic Response," *Asia Pacific Journal of Clinical Nutrition* 24, no. 4 (2015): 620–625, https://doi.org/10.6133/apjcn.2015.24.4.13.

5. M. Leeman, E. Ostman, and I. Björck, "Vinegar Dressing and Cold Storage of Potatoes Lowers Postprandial Glycaemic and Insulinaemic Responses in Healthy Subjects," *European Journal of Clinical Nutrition* 59, no. 11 (November 2005):1266–1271, https://doi.org/10.1038/sj.ejcn.1602238.

6. Kitt Falk Petersen, Sylvie Dufour, David B. Savage, Stefan Bilz, Gina Solomon, Shin Yonemitsu, Gary W. Cline, et al., "The Role of Skeletal Muscle Insulin Resistance in the Pathogenesis of the Metabolic Syndrome," *Proceedings of the National Academy of Sciences* 104, no. 31 (July 2007): 12587–12594, https://doi.org/10.1073/pnas.0705408104.

7. Stuart M. Phillips, Douglas Paddon-Jones, and Donald K. Layman, "Optimizing Adult Protein Intake during Catabolic Health Conditions," *Advances in Nutrition* 11, no. 4 (2020): S1058–S1069, https://doi.org/10.1093/advances/nmaa047.

8. Maximilian Andreas Storz and Alvaro Luis Ronco, "Nutrient Intake in Low-Carbohydrate Diets in Comparison to the 2020–2025 Dietary Guidelines for Americans: A Cross-Sectional Study," *British Journal of Nutrition* 129, no. 6 (2023): 1023–1036, https://doi.org/10.1017/S0007114522001908.

9. Mark Cucuzzella, Adele Hite, Kaitlyn Patterson, Laura Saslow, and Rory Heath, "A Clinician's Guide to Inpatient Low-Carbohydrate Diets for Remission of Type 2 Diabetes: Toward a Standard of Care Protocol," *Diabetes Management* 9, no. 1 (2019): 7–19.

10. Paula Byrne, Maryanne Demasi, Mark Jones, Susan M. Smith, Kirsty K. O'Brien, and Robert DuBroff, "Evaluating the Association between Low-Density Lipoprotein Cholesterol Reduction and Relative and Absolute Effects of Statin Treatment: A Systematic Review and Meta-analysis," *JAMA Internal Medicine* 182, no. 5 (May 2022): 474–481, https://doi.org/10.1001/jamainternmed.2022.0134.

11. Cara B. Ebbeling, Janis F. Swain, Henry A. Feldman, William W. Wong, David L. Hachey, Erica Garcia-Lago, and David S. Ludwig, "Effects of Dietary Composition on Energy Expenditure during Weight-Loss Maintenance," *JAMA* 307, no. 24 (2012): 2627–2634, https://doi.org/10.1001/jama.2012.6607.

12. Andrew P. DeFilippis and Laurence S. Sperling, "Understanding Omega-3's," *American Heart Journal* 151, no. 3 (March 2006): 564–570, https://doi.org/10.1016/j.ahj.2005.03.051.

13. Chris McGlory, Philip C. Calder, and Everson A. Nunes, "The Influence of Omega-3 Fatty Acids on Skeletal Muscle Protein Turnover in Health, Disuse, and Disease," *Frontiers in Nutrition* 6 (August 2019), https://doi.org/10.3389/fnut.2019.00144.

14. Artemis Simopoulos, "An Increase in the Omega-6/Omega-3 Fatty Acid Ratio Increases the Risk for Obesity," *Nutrients* 8, no. 3 (March 2016): 128, https://doi.org/10.3390/nu8030128.

15. Frank M. Sacks, Alice H. Lichtenstein, Jason H. Y. Wu, Lawrence J. Appel, Mark A. Creager, Penny M. Kris-Etherton, Michael Miller, et al., "Dietary Fats and Cardiovascular Disease: A Presidential Advisory from the American Heart Association," *Circulation* 136, no. 3 (July 2017), https://doi.org/10.1161/cir.0000000000000510.

16. R. Micha, J. L. Peñalvo, F. Cudhea, F. Imamura, C. D. Rehm, and D. Mozaffarian, "Association between Dietary Factors and Mortality from Heart Disease, Stroke, and Type 2 Diabetes in the United States," *JAMA* 317, no. 9 (2017): 912–924, https://doi.org/10.1001/jama.2017.0947.

17. Gay Hendricks, *The Big Leap: Conquer Your Hidden Fear and Take Life to the Next Level* (New York: HarperCollins, 2010).

CHAPTER 7: THE LYON PROTOCOL MEAL PLANS

1. Alex Leaf and Jose Antonio, "The Effects of Overfeeding on Body Composition: The Role of Macronutrient Composition—A Narrative Review," *International Journal of Exercise Science* 10, no. 8 (December 2017).

2. Leroy et al., "Animal Board Invited Review."

3. A. P. Simopoulos, H. A. Norman, and J. E. Gillaspy, "Purslane in Human Nutrition and Its Potential for World Agriculture," *World Review of Nutrition and Dietetics* 77 (1995): 47–74, https://doi.org/10.1159/000424465.

4. T. van Vliet and M. B. Katan, "Lower Ratio of N-3 to N-6 Fatty Acids in Cultured Than in Wild Fish," *American Journal of Clinical Nutrition* 51, no. 1 (January 1990): 1–2, https://doi.org/10.1093/ajcn/51.1.1.

5. A. P. Simopoulos and N. Salem, "Egg Yolk as a Source of Long-Chain Polyunsaturated Fatty Acids in Infant Feeding," *American Journal of Clinical Nutrition* 55, no. 2 (February 1992): 411–414, https://doi.org/10.1093/ajcn/55 .2.411.

6. Stuart M. Phillips, Stéphanie Chevalier, and Heather J. Leidy, "Protein 'Requirements' beyond the RDA: Implications for Optimizing Health," *Applied Physiology, Nutrition, and Metabolism* 41, no. 5 (May 2016): 565–572, https:// doi.org/10.1139/apnm-2015-0550.

7. Juergen Bauer, Gianni Biolo, Tommy Cederholm, Matteo Cesari, Alfonso Cruz-Jentoft, John Morley, Stuart Phillips, Cornel Sieber, Peter Stehle, Daniel Teta, Renuka Visvanathan, Elena Volpi, and Yves Boirie, "Evidence-Based Recommendations for Optimal Dietary Protein Intake in Older People: A Position Paper from the PROT-AGE Study Group," *Journal of the American Medical Directors Association* 14 (2013), https://doi.org/10.1016/j.jamda .2013.05.021.

8. R. Jäger, C. M. Kerksick, B. I. Campbell, P. J. Cribb, S. D. Wells, T. M. Skwiat, M. Purpura, T. N. Ziegenfuss, A. A. Ferrando, S. M. Arent, A. E. Smith-Ryan, J. R. Stout, P. J. Arciero, M. J. Ormsbee, L. W. Taylor, C. D. Wilborn, D. S. Kalman, R. B. Kreider, D. S. Willoughby, J. R. Hoffman, and J. Antonio, "International Society of Sports Nutrition Position Stand: Protein and Exercise," *Journal of the International Society of Sports Nutrition* 14, no. 20 (2017), https:// doi.org/10.1186/s12970-017-0177-8.

9. Eric R. Helms, Alan A. Aragon, and Peter J. Fitschen, "Evidence-Based Recommendations for Natural Bodybuilding Contest Preparation: Nutrition and Supplementation," *Journal of the International Society of Sports Nutrition* 11, no. 1 (August 2014), https://doi.org/10.1186/1550-2783-11-20.

10. Helms et al., "Evidence-Based Recommendations."

11. Chad M. Kerksick, Shawn Arent, Brad J. Schoenfeld, Jeffrey R. Stout, Bill Campbell, Colin D. Wilborn, Lem Taylor, et al., "International Society of Sports Nutrition Position Stand: Nutrient Timing," *Journal of the International Society of Sports Nutrition* 14, no. 1 (August 2017), https://doi.org/10.1186/s12970-017 -0189-4.

12. Abdullah Alghannam, Javier Gonzalez, and James Betts, "Restoration of Muscle Glycogen and Functional Capacity: Role of Post-Exercise Carbohydrate and Protein Co-Ingestion," *Nutrients* 10, no. 2 (February 2018): 253, https:// doi.org/10.3390/nu10020253.

13. Matthew Morrison, Shona L. Halson, Jonathon Weakley, and John A. Hawley, "Sleep, Circadian Biology and Skeletal Muscle Interactions: Implications for

Metabolic Health," *Sleep Medicine Reviews* 66 (December 2022): 101700, https://doi.org/10.1016/j.smrv.2022.101700.

14. Alan Aragon, Flexible Dieting: *A Science-Based, Reality-Tested Method for Achieving and Maintaining Your Optimal Physique, Performance and Health* (Las Vegas, NV: Victory Belt Publishing, 2022).

CHAPTER 8: BASELINE ASSESSMENT: WHERE ARE YOU AT?

1. Assessing Your Weight and Health Risk," National Heart, Lung, and Blood Institute, National Institutes of Health, accessed May 2, 2023, https://www.nhlbi.nih.gov/health/educational/lose_wt/risk.htm.

2. "Assessing Your Weight and Health Risk."

3. R. Ross, I. J. Neeland, S. Yamashita, et al., "Waist Circumference as a Vital Sign in Clinical Practice: A Consensus Statement from the IAS and ICCR Working Group on Visceral Obesity," *Nature Reviews Endocrinology* 16 (February 2020): 177–189, https://doi.org/10.1038/s41574-019-0310-7.

4. Ross et al., "Waist Circumference."

5. M. Ashwell, P. Gunn, and S. Gibson, "Waist-to-Height Ratio Is a Better Screening Tool Than Waist Circumference and BMI for Adult Cardiometabolic Risk Factors: Systematic Review and Meta-Analysis," *Obesity Reviews* 13, no. 3 (March 2012): 275–286, https://doi.org/10.1111/j.1467-789X.2011.00952.x.

6. Margaret Ashwell and Sigrid Gibson, "Waist-to-Height Ratio as an Indicator of 'Early Health Risk': Simpler and More Predictive Than Using a 'Matrix' Based on BMI and Waist Circumference," *BMJ Open* 6, no. 3 (2016): e010159, https://doi.org/10.1136/bmjopen-2015-010159.

7. Richard A. Dickey, D. Bartuska, George W. Bray, C. Wayne Callaway, Eugene T. Davidson, Stanley Feld, Robert T. Ferraro, et al., "AACE/ACE Position Statement on the Prevention, Diagnosis, and Treatment of Obesity (1998 Revision)," *Endocrine Practice* 4, no. 5 (1998): 297–350.

8. Fanny Buckinx, Francesco Landi, Matteo Cesari, Roger A. Fielding, Marjolein Visser, Klaus Engelke, Stefania Maggi, et al., "Pitfalls in the Measurement of Muscle Mass: A Need for a Reference Standard," *Journal of Cachexia, Sarcopenia and Muscle* 9, no. 2 (January 2018): 269–278, https://doi.org/10.1002/jcsm.12268.

9. M. A. Czeck, C. J. Raymond-Pope, P. R. Stanforth, A. Carbuhn, T. A. Bosch, C. W. Bach, J. M. Oliver, and D. R. Dengel, "Total and Regional Body Composition of NCAA Division I Collegiate Female Softball Athletes," *International Journal of Sports Medicine* 40, no. 10 (September 2019): 645–649, https://doi.org/10.1055/a-0962-1283; T. A. Bosch, A. F. Carbuhn, P. R. Stanforth, J. M. Oliver, K. A. Keller, and D. R. Dengel, "Body Composition and Bone Mineral Density of Division 1 Collegiate Football Players: A Consortium of College Athlete Research Study," *Journal of Strength and*

Conditioning Research 33, no. 5 (May 2019): 1339–1346, https://doi.org/10.1519 /JSC.0000000000001888; K. Y. Cheng, S. K. Chow, V. W. Hung, C. H. Wong, R. M. Wong, C. S. Tsang, T. Kwok, and W. H. Cheung, "Diagnosis of Sarcopenia by Evaluating Skeletal Muscle Mass by Adjusted Bioimpedance Analysis Validated with Dual-Energy X-ray Absorptiometry," *Journal of Cachexia, Sarcopenia and Muscle* 12, no. 6 (December 2021): 2163–2173, https://doi .org/10.1002/jcsm.12825; R. N. Baumgartner, K. M. Koehler, D. Gallagher, L. Romero, S. B. Heymsfield, R. R. Ross, P. J. Garry, and R. D. Lindeman, "Epidemiology of Sarcopenia among the Elderly in New Mexico," *American Journal of Epidemiology* 147, no. 8 (April 1998): 755–763, https://doi .org/10.1093/oxfordjournals.aje.a009520, erratum in *American Journal of Epidemiology* 149, no. 12 (June 1999):1161.; D. Gallagher, M. Visser, R. E. De Meersman, D. Sepúlveda, R. N. Baumgartner, R. N. Pierson, T. Harris, and S. B. Heymsfield, "Appendicular Skeletal Muscle Mass: Effects of Age, Gender, and Ethnicity," *Journal of Applied Physiology* 83, no. 1 (July 1997): 229–239, https://doi.org/10.1152/jappl.1997.83.1.229

10. Pablo Esteban Morales, Jose Luis Bucarey, and Alejandra Espinosa, "Muscle Lipid Metabolism: Role of Lipid Droplets and Perilipins," *Journal of Diabetes Research* 2017 (June 2017): 1–10, https://doi.org/10.1155/2017/1789395.

11. William E. Kraus, Joseph A. Houmard, Brian D. Duscha, Kenneth J. Knetzger, Michelle B. Wharton, Jennifer S. McCartney, Connie W. Bales, et al., "Effects of the Amount and Intensity of Exercise on Plasma Lipoproteins," *New England Journal of Medicine* 347, no. 19 (November 2002): 1483–1492, https://doi.org/10 .1056/nejmoa020194.

12. "Causes of High Cholesterol," American Heart Association, https:// www.heart.org/en/health-topics/cholesterol/causes-of-high-cholesterol.

13. Gina Wood, Anna Murrell, Tom van der Touw, and Neil Smart, "HIIT Is Not Superior to MICT in Altering Blood Lipids: A Systematic Review and Meta-Analysis," *BMJ Open Sport & Exercise Medicine* 5, no. 1 (December 2019), https:// doi.org/10.1136/bmjsem-2019-000647.

14. David J. Jenkins, "Effects of a Dietary Portfolio of Cholesterol-Lowering Foods vs. Lovastatin on Serum Lipids and C-Reactive Protein," *JAMA* 290, no. 4 (July 2003): 502, https://doi.org/10.1001/jama.290.4.502.

15. Giuseppe Pilia, Wei-Min Chen, Angelo Scuteri, Marco Orrú, Giuseppe Albai, Mariano Dei, Sandra Lai, et al., "Heritability of Cardiovascular and Personality Traits in 6,148 Sardinians," *PLOS Genetics* 2, no. 8 (August 2006), https://doi.org /10.1371/journal.pgen.0020132.

16. Elisa Fabbrini, Shelby Sullivan, and Samuel Klein, "Obesity and Nonalcoholic Fatty Liver Disease: Biochemical, Metabolic, and Clinical Implications," *Hepatology* 51, no. 2 (February 2009): 679–689, https://doi.org/10.1002/hep .23280.

17. Christoph Gasteyger, Thomas Meinert Larsen, Frank Vercruysse, and Arne Astrup, "Effect of a Dietary-Induced Weight Loss on Liver Enzymes in Obese Subjects," *American Journal of Clinical Nutrition* 87, no. 5 (May 2008): 1141–1147, https://doi.org/10.1093/ajcn/87.5.1141.

18. Jaimy Villavicencio Kim, and George Y. Wu, "Body Building and Aminotransferase Elevations: A Review," *Journal of Clinical and Translational Hepatology* 8, no. 2 (2020): 161, https://doi.org/10.14218/JCTH.2020.00005.

19. Omair Yousuf, Bibhu D. Mohanty, Seth S. Martin, Parag H. Joshi, Michael J. Blaha, Khurram Nasir, Roger S. Blumenthal, and Matthew J. Budoff, "High-Sensitivity C-Reactive Protein and Cardiovascular Disease," *Journal of the American College of Cardiology* 62, no. 5 (July 2013): 397–408, https://doi.org/10.1016/j.jacc.2013.05.016.

20. Shari S. Bassuk, Nader Rifai, and Paul M. Ridker, "High-Sensitivity C-Reactive Protein," *Current Problems in Cardiology* 29, no. 8 (August 2004): 439–493, https://doi.org/10.1016/j.cpcardiol.2004.03.004.

21. Yousuf et al., "High-Sensitivity C-Reactive Protein."

22. Joseph W. Beals, Nicholas A. Burd, Daniel R. Moore, and Stephan van Vliet, "Obesity Alters the Muscle Protein Synthetic Response to Nutrition and Exercise," *Frontiers in Nutrition* 6 (June 2019), https://doi.org/10.3389/fnut.2019.00087.

23. Paul M. Ridker, "The Jupiter Trial," *Circulation: Cardiovascular Quality and Outcomes* 2, no. 3 (August 2009): 279–285, https://doi.org/10.1161/circoutcomes.109.868299.

24. "Blood Glucose (Sugar) Test," Cleveland Clinic, https://my.clevelandclinic.org/health/diagnostics/12363-blood-glucose-test.

25. Melissa L. Erickson, Nathan T. Jenkins, and Kevin K. McCully, "Exercise after You Eat: Hitting the Postprandial Glucose Target," *Frontiers in Endocrinology* 8 (September 2017), https://doi.org/10.3389/fendo.2017.00228.

26. Lluis Campins, Marcella Camps, Ariadna Riera, Eulogio Pleguezuelos, Juan Carlos Yebenes, and Mateu Serra-Prat, "Oral Drugs Related with Muscle Wasting and Sarcopenia: A Review," *Pharmacology* 99, nos. 1–2 (August 2016): 1–8, https://doi.org/10.1159/000448247.

27. Edward R. Laskowski, "What's a Normal Resting Heart Rate?" Mayo Clinic, https://www.mayoclinic.org/healthy-lifestyle/fitness/expert-answers/heart-rate/faq-20057979.

CHAPTER 9: TRAINING: THE MINIMUM EFFECTIVE DOSE TO ACHIEVE THE MAXIMUM RESULT

1. Jinger S. Gottschall, Joshua J. Davis, Bryce Hastings, and Heather J. Porter, "Exercise Time and Intensity: How Much Is Too Much?" *International Journal of*

Sports Physiology and Performance 15, no. 6 (February 2020): 808–815, https://doi
.org/10.1123/ijspp.2019-0208.

2. Jozo Grgic, Luke C. McIlvenna, Jackson J. Fyfe, Filip Sabol, David J. Bishop,
    Brad J. Schoenfeld, and Zeljko Pedisic, "Does Aerobic Training Promote the
    Same Skeletal Muscle Hypertrophy as Resistance Training? A Systematic Review
    and Meta-Analysis," *Sports Medicine* 49, no. 2 (October 2018): 233–254, https://
    doi.org/10.1007/s40279-018-1008-z.

3. Gottschall et al., "Exercise Time and Intensity."

4. Gottschall et al., "Exercise Time and Intensity."

5. Brian G. Sutton, *NASM Essentials of Personal Fitness Training* (Burlington, MA:
    Jones & Bartlett Learning, 2022).

6. Julien Robineau, Nicolas Babault, Julien Piscione, Mathieu Lacome, and André
    X. Bigard, "Specific Training Effects of Concurrent Aerobic and Strength
    Exercises Depend on Recovery Duration," *Journal of Strength and Conditioning
    Research* 30, no. 3 (March 2016): 672–683, https://doi.org/10.1519/jsc
    .0000000000000798.

7. Paul T. Reidy, Ziad S. Mahmassani, Alec I. McKenzie, Jonathan J. Petrocelli,
    Scott A. Summers, and Micah J. Drummond, "Influence of Exercise Training on
    Skeletal Muscle Insulin Resistance in Aging: Spotlight on Muscle Ceramides,"
    International Journal of Molecular Sciences 21, no. 4 (February 2020): 1514,
    https://doi.org/10.3390/ijms21041514.

8. Kelly McGonigal, *The Upside of Stress: Why Stress Is Good for You, and How to Get
    Good at It* (New York: Avery, 2016).

INDEX

ABOUT THE AUTHOR

DR. GABRIELLE LYON is a board-certified family physician who completed a combined research and clinical fellowship in geriatrics and nutritional sciences at Washington University in St. Louis. She completed her undergraduate training in nutritional sciences at the University of Illinois. Dr. Lyon is a subject-matter expert and educator in the practical application of protein types and levels for health, performance, aging, and disease prevention. She has continued to receive mentorship from Donald Layman, PhD, over the course of two decades to help bring protein metabolism and nutrition from the bench to the bedside. Find out more at drgabriellelyon.com.